More Praise for *Yoga for Depression*

"Amy Weintraub's work is some of the most important in our world today for helping humanity understand more deeply the significance of the mind-body connection. Her insights are inspirational for yoga teachers and all readers. Her in-depth understanding of her subject is an important basis for personal as well as societal transformation."

—RAMA JYOTI VERNON, founder,
American Yoga College

"In the compassionate voice of someone who definitely knows the territory of depression, Amy Weintraub presents Yoga science and personal stories, research results and poetry, and practice instructions that are genuinely interesting in this very readable book that is both comprehensive and totally inspiring."

—SYLVIA BOORSTEIN, author of
That's Funny You Don't Look Like a Buddhist and
It's Easier Than You Think: The Buddhist Way to Happiness

"This is truly a beautifully written encyclopedia of yoga for depression. It is rare to find such a generous soul, willing to embrace all approaches to yoga, unbiased and yet having intelligent discernment and advice for those searching for help. Amy offers many guidelines and solutions through yoga, to both those who suffer from depression and to yoga teachers working with them."

—ANGELA FARMER, internationally known yoga teacher
and creator of *The Feminine Unfolding* video

"With clarity, compassion, and the courage of a person who has lived her own story all the way through, Amy Weintraub offers readers a self-aware, self-creating path through the darker thickets of a life. Her specific, gracefully presented suggestions for joining breath, body, movement, and mind bring one of the great wisdom traditions into a newly useful context, an essential means for renewing and reawakening contemporary life."

—JANE HIRSHFIELD, author of five books of poetry,
most recently *Given Sugar, Given Salt: Poems*

"Amy Weintraub is a gifted teacher whose clarity and warmth I have admired for years, but it wasn't until I read this book that I understood the genesis of her profound emotional connection to yoga. Amy has personally made the journey from the darkness of depression to the light of full aliveness. The value of this kind of personal experience in a yoga teacher cannot be overestimated, and it jumps off the pages of this book. If you are looking for an inspiring and trustworthy guide to heal into a whole new life, look no further."

—RICHARD FAULDS, M.A., J.D., senior Kripalu teacher
and author of the forthcoming
Kripalu Yoga: A Guide to Practice On and Off the Mat

"Yoga philosophy describes our true nature as free, radiant, and vibrant. In a clear, direct, and grounded approach, this brilliant and comprehensive book offers guideposts for those seeking to reclaim their birthright of joy."

—SUDHIR JONATHAN FOUST, president,
Kripalu Center for Yoga and Health

"Amy Weintraub's *Yoga for Depression* offers us a powerful and comprehensive guidebook that provides the reader with a precise path for healing from depression. Her penetrating insights are derived with the precision of someone who has traversed the intricate path of healing from depression and has come back to show us the way to our own healing. Amy has experienced the simple truth that yoga works because it offers a comprehensive approach to healing. She has discovered the timeless teachings of yoga that don't ask us to believe or depend upon someone else's authority. Yoga puts us squarely in the driver's seat and shows us how to heal our self. Yoga is a set of applied tools that support us in living, pure and simply, a life that is free of suffering. This book belongs in the hands of every person who experiences depression and in the library of every therapist who works with people suffering from depression."

—RICHARD C. MILLER, PH.D., clinical psychologist,
teacher of Advaitayana Yoga, co-founder of the International
Association of Yoga Therapy, and founding editor of *The Professional
Journal of the International Association of Yoga Therapy*

yoga for depression

yoga for depression

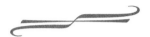

a compassionate guide to
relieve suffering through yoga

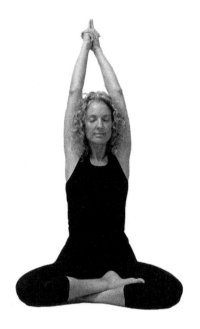

AMY WEINTRAUB

Foreword by Stephen Cope, LICSW
Preface by Richard Brown, M.D.

BROADWAY BOOKS ～ *new york*

BROADWAY

Yoga for Depression. Copyright © 2004 by Amy Weintraub. All rights reserved. No part of this book may be reproduced or transmitted in any form or by any means, electronic or mechanical, including photocopying, recording, or by any information storage and retrieval system, without written permission from the publisher. For information, address Broadway Books, a division of Random House, Inc.

PRINTED IN THE UNITED STATES OF AMERICA

BROADWAY BOOKS and its logo, a letter B bisected on the diagonal, are trademarks of Random House, Inc.

Visit our website at www.broadwaybooks.com.

First edition published 2004.

Book design by Erin L. Matherne and Tina Thompson
Photographs by Léo A. Gosselin and Judith Belsham Singer
Digital photo production by Judith Belsham Singer

Library of Congress Cataloging-in-Publication Data

Weintraub, Amy.
    Yoga for depression : a compassionate guide to relieve suffering through Yoga /
Amy Weintraub ; with forewords by Stephen Cope and Richard Brown.
        p. cm.
    Includes bibliographical references.
    ISBN 0-7679-1450-3
    1. Depression, Mental—Alternative treatment—Popular works. 2. Yoga—Psychological aspects—Popular works. 3. Yoga. I. Title.

RC537.W347 2004
616.85'27'06—dc21   2003052203

20 19 18 17 16 15 14

In celebration of the one who reminds me that we always have a choice,
my daughter, Marlana Ruth Droz.
And to the one I choose.

Crying is one of the highest devotional songs. One who knows crying, knows spiritual practice. If you can cry with a pure heart, nothing else compares to such a prayer. Crying includes all the principles of Yoga.

—SWAMI KRIPALU[I]

CONTENTS

by Stephen Cope

Depression appears to be a universal human experience. We are fortunate, then, to live in a time when being depressed no longer marks us as flawed, or possessed, or sinful—or even separate from God. Depression marks us only as human. We are, as Kierkegaard said, "the animal who suffers."

But what *is* this particular suffering of depression? The conventional wisdom holds depression to be a mood disorder: "I'm depressed. I'm out of sorts. I'm sad." But I think most of us know that it's a much more complicated animal. It shows up in vastly different ways—not just as a bleak mood. It shows up in our self-defeating and addictive behaviors. It shows up in our thoughts as negative self-talk. It shows up in the very way we perceive ourselves, others, and the world. It even shows up in the health of our immune functioning.

No, depression is not just a mood disorder. Oftentimes when we're depressed, in fact, we don't even *feel* depressed. Indeed, we may feel little of anything at all. Most of us know this territory, don't we? Moving through life as in a trance? "It's too painful to look. Too painful to feel." We run to the TV, or for a pint of ice cream, or to the mall. How can we shut life out? In fact, this experience of alienation from life is really the heart of depression. *Depression manifests as our inability to be present for the experience of life.* At its root, depression signals a difficulty with Being itself.

Emily Dickinson, who wrestled magnificently with depression, got the tone of this suffering just right:

> There is a pain—so utter—
> It swallows substance up—
> Then covers the Abyss with Trance—
> So Memory can step
> Around—across—upon it—

As one within a Swoon
Goes safely—Where an open eye—
Would drop him—Bone by Bone.

Let's face it: Life is sometimes almost too difficult to bear. And so most of us spend some part of our energy avoiding Being—avoiding the anxiety, the pain, the sheer sensation of it all. And in these times we may enter the trance of depression about which Dickinson writes.

Because we've studied depression so intently over the past two decades, we now know that many of us live most of our lives mildly depressed. Separated—if you will—from our own (dare I say it?) Life Force. Afraid of really living, we make deals with ourselves in order not to feel, not to live. We make compromises that keep us at arm's length from life—secluded from the raw ups and downs of being human. Psychologists may call these deals pathological solutions. They may show up over time as "symptoms."

But there is good news! It turns out that *the wish to be* also marks us as human. The wish to live fully—even in the face of certain death. In fact, for some of us, the effort to become fully alive may be more important than survival itself. Most of us long to give up our compromises and our deals, to be fully present for the experience of life. But how can we do it? How can we learn to bear what Jon Kabat Zinn called the "full catastrophe of life"? Is psychotherapy enough? Are pills enough?

Emily Dickinson wrote poetry in order to live. For her, art was medicine—and taking a daily dose was literally a life-or-death affair. What do *we* do to wrestle with our problems with Being? What medicine do we take? For medicine, of some kind, I think, will be required.

In recent years, many in the West have found that the Eastern contemplative traditions—and particularly Yoga—speak directly to these problems of Being. What a surprise! We have discovered that the Yoga traditions were interested precisely in the problem of ordinary human suffering and misery. What are its root causes? What are its antidotes?

Yogis, practicing primarily on the Indian subcontinent over the course of literally thousands of years, explored every aspect of human suffering—physical, mental, behavioral, emotional, and spiritual. They became experts—not just at palliation but at pulling up suffering by its roots.

The Yoga traditions developed a very different point of view about suffering than have Western psychological traditions. Their investigations led them to believe that any of us who are not living up to our potential, who are not living fully, are in some fashion depressed. The Yoga traditions came to place a great value on development. This tradition sees the self as a kind of "seed" with unlimited potential—a river of energy, intelligence, and consciousness. They believed that unless you're creating the right conditions for the sprouting of this auspicious and fulsome seed—if you're not living fully—you *will* be in some fashion depressed. As a friend of mine used to say: "If you ain't livin', honey, you dyin.'"

And how do we live? Is there help here in the Yoga traditions? There is indeed. The central archetype of the Yoga tradition is the *jivan mukti*—the "soul awake in this life." Literally, "living liberation." Yoga itself is the complex science of awakening to who we are, who we *can be*. Yogis believed that we can create our own lives, our own happiness. How we live each moment actually creates our experience of life. Yogis get very concrete about this. How we move, breathe, eat, bathe, sleep, dream, and think all create our experience of the moment. There is an enormous amount of very practical help in the Yogic traditions: how to live fully! The jivan mukti!

In this book, Amy Weintraub directly addresses the core of depression: the problem of Being itself, in the finest tradition of Yoga. *Yoga for Depression* is an astonishingly comprehensive guide to the art and science of Yoga. In these pages, Amy gives us enormous amounts of very detailed, practical, concrete tools. Her suggestions for how Yoga can help overcome depression are based on her thorough research, her conversations with a wide range of major American and world teachers, and her own experience as both a student of Yoga and a senior Kripalu teacher and mentor. And there is so much heart in this book. Amy tells inspiring and beautifully written stories of real practice—her own, her colleagues', and her students'.

This book is both a "how to" and a "why bother" rolled into one. But its message is much bigger than "how to" practice Yoga. Amy writes her way through the obstacles, her own and ours too, that keep us from living fully. Herein lies a Yogic blueprint for how to be a human being, written by a compassionate and generous teacher.

What makes Amy's book particularly noble is that she speaks directly from her own experience. To our great fortune, she has woven in her own personal story—the story of one human being's wrestling with Being itself. As we read, we begin to understand her astonishing recovery from depression. Like Amy herself, who spent several months as scholar-in-residence at Kripalu Center, this book vibrates with life.

The great thing about the Yoga traditions is that they don't give us any one particular way to be. They give us something much more precious: a way to find out directly and to know incontrovertibly who we already Are. Amy's book is an important contribution to the best spirit of this path in America and the world.

Stephen Cope, LICSW, is senior scholar-in-residence at Kripalu Center, Lenox, MA, and author of Yoga and the Quest for the True Self.

by Richard Brown

Depression is a worldwide epidemic. It is the leading illness in adults and often occurs with other serious illnesses, such as heart disease, stroke, and arthritis. It predisposes sufferers to Alzheimer's and Parkinson's diseases, and accelerates aging of the body and brain. In the United States, we have an unprecedented rise in the rates of child and teen suicide. The depression epidemic is even worse in developing countries and will increase as people live longer. Women and older people have an increased risk of depression.

What causes depression? In mainstream medicine, it is believed to be an overactivation of the stress-response part of the nervous system. Recent evidence indicates it is also associated with underactivation of the well-being (parasympathetic) part of the nervous system.

The current medical treatment of depression predominantly focuses on antidepressants, which calm the stress-response system. This approach has numerous drawbacks. Antidepressants have immediate side effects. Consequently, many people are reluctant to start medication or become unwilling to continue it for more than three months. The lack of any solid data on the long-term side effects of antidepressants is a growing concern. Furthermore, prescription antidepressants are costly. People without prescription insurance coverage and those living in less industrialized countries cannot afford to see doctors or to pay for these medications. Surprisingly, even in Australia, the socialized health service budget for medication is projected to go bankrupt by 2005, primarily because of the cost of antidepressants and secondarily the cost of arthritis drugs.

Finally, what I have seen so often is that medication reduces the desperation and suicidality that the depressed person feels, but it does not touch the whole being. It does not bring out the feelings of joy and love inside all of us. Five years ago, while speaking at a United Nations symposium on natural treatments for worldwide depression, I discovered a wealth of medical and psychiatric research on how Yoga breathing and other Yoga practices effectively relieve depression. Since then, I have trained to bring these healing techniques to a wide range of people, including patients and health care providers, who suffer from stress and depression.

I met Amy in the course of her research for this book, and was impressed by her loving spirit and depth of character. In this book she describes from her own experience and that of others how to use the eight limbs of Yoga to overcome depression. Yoga offers an alternative to the problems of conventional medical treatment for depression. It does not have detrimental side effects; it has side *benefits* for the body and mind. It is extremely cost effective and can be taught to large groups. Yoga practices address the root cause of depression: the energy drain caused by the overreactions of our mind to the stresses of our world and the pressures of our own fears and desires. By activating our innate mental, physical, and spiritual healing capacities, Yoga practice strengthens our feelings of joy, peace, and connectedness.

To establish an effective Yoga practice requires discipline, commitment, and time. These are the greatest impediments, but only through effort and commitment can we hope to grow. The choice is yours.

Reading about Yoga is the first step. The next step is experiencing Yoga under the guidance of a skilled teacher. This book is your map to finding the right teacher and the best practices to help you heal yourself. Read it and apply the practices to your daily life.

Richard P. Brown, M.D., is associate professor of clinical psychiatry at Columbia University College of Physicians and Surgeons, New York, NY, and co-author of Stop Depression Now: SAM-E.

empty pockets

Know that God loves empty hands.

—WERNER BERGENGRUEN, from "The Art of Heavenly Accounting"

Essence is emptiness.
Everything else, accidental.

Emptiness brings peace to your loving.
Everything else, disease.

In this world of trickery emptiness
Is what your soul wants.

—RUMI, from "The Pattern Improves"[1]

November in coastal New England is a time to gather with friends in front of the fire. It's a wonderful month to sit before the computer and finish that assignment, write a long e-mail to a faraway friend, or curl up in your favorite chair with a good novel. But if you're feeling depressed, you may not have the energy or the will to do any of these things. For the sixteen years I lived there, November in New England was my low point, the time when my chronic depression came into full bloom, fertilized by heavy cloud cover and rain. There were few temptingly warm days to break the bleak monotony of life lived indoors, and dawn broke without a glimpse of the sun.

On just such a damp, gray November afternoon, the tail end of hurricane season in 1985, I sat on my psychiatrist's couch in Providence, Rhode Island, feeling a familiar sense of emptiness. I didn't suffer in the way Virginia Woolf made famous, with "wave after wave of agony." Depression for me was, as Emily Dickinson describes it, "an element of blank." A stultifying numbness had settled in. Sometimes I rose in the morning with what felt like a layer of cotton batting between my brain and my cranium. Neither coffee nor exercise penetrated the thickening. I moved as though through a fog. My senses were dulled and my perceptions impaired. One day, I sent a check to our health insurance carrier for the entire checking account balance, instead of the payment due. I forgot important meetings. I lost keys, gloves, and once, even my car in a parking lot.

Only a few weeks before, my partner and I had spent a frantic morning in high wind, nailing plywood over the long Victorian windows of our Newport home. Hurricane Gloria was traveling up the coast, and the weather service was predicting winds of 125 miles per hour and torrential rain for later that afternoon. Outside, we pushed large potted plants against the protection of the garden walls, tied back the wisteria, carried outdoor furniture and hanging baskets of dead geraniums into the basement, and worried about the creaking limb of the hundred-year-old beech tree that hung over the roof. I say "we," but the truth was, I hadn't been much help. Tasks that I performed automatically when I was well were suddenly impossible. I had forgotten how to stack the chairs and fold the chaise longue, and I kept dropping the hammer and nails into the rhododendron bushes. Neither my partner's threats and curses—*Damn it, Amy, pay attention! Look what you're doing!*—nor the electron-charged wind in which we worked could blow the fog from my brain, a fog that was to linger four more years.

Several weeks later, I sat on my therapist's couch, telling her that my life was meaningless. How could I justify my existence when my novels were stacking up, unpublished, in my closet? "You're one of those people who will always have empty pockets," she said. And I visualized myself, like Virginia Woolf, filling those empty pockets with stones and stepping into the river.

Until I took my first Yoga class at Kripalu Center in Lenox, Massachusetts, I believed my psychiatrist was right. My empty pockets and my need for antidepressant medication felt like a life sentence. In that first class, the instructor had us place our hands in prayer position in front of our hearts. "Take a deep breath in," she said, "and fill your heart with light. Hold the breath and feel the light as healing energy expand through your chest and through your whole body. Exhale and open your palms to receive. Stay empty. God loves your empty hands."

And right there, in that moment, I realized that there was another way to see my depression. "Empty pockets" wasn't a curse but a blessing. I had more room for the divine inside me. This new insight didn't blow the fog of depression from my mind. It simply opened a window through which I saw the possibility of feeling better, the possibility of extending, through the rest of my day, the good feeling I had in those moments after Yoga class. In those moments I felt alive, not just in my mind, which at that moment was perceiving how good I felt, not just in my belly, rumbling with hunger, not just in my heart, expanding with love, but down into my fingertips, up to the crown of my head, and down into my toes. Every cell felt awake and in a state of awe, a state beyond happiness in which I felt connected to all beings.

Might it be possible to feel this more in my life? I wondered. To live from this awakened state? Even as I folded my blanket into the cupboard and put my cushion away, I was beginning to doubt my own experience of happiness. "But I am one of those people with empty pockets. A depressed person. I don't deserve to be happy." I had come right back to the nearly constant river of negative self-talk that flowed so steadily through my mind. Still, though, my body felt better than it had before the class, and as I walked down the wide corridor to the dining chapel for breakfast, I could feel the easy smile on my face. Not a social mask, the smile seemed to rise up from beneath the surface, creating a little island of peace in the stream of my negativity.

I had come to Kripalu Center because I had found a Kripalu catalogue in my absent friend's mailbox when I collected her mail. I lived less than three hours away but had never heard of the place. Though I'd practiced Yoga from time to time, between rounds of meditation during Transcendental Meditation retreats in the early seventies and on my own with the scratchy Richard Hittleman records I bought secondhand, I did not have a regular practice and had never taken a Yoga class. So I registered for a few days in the Rest and Renewal program, which is a little less structured than other Kripalu programs. There were morning workshops taught by a variety of teachers, morning and afternoon Yoga classes, evening programs of music and chanting, and free afternoons. With my free time, I walked the lovely grounds and I perused the bookstore, buying my first books about Yoga practice and philosophy and a few audiotapes with Yoga sequences led by Kripalu teachers.

When I returned to Newport, I began to get up a little earlier. First thing in the morning, I would push the play button on my boom box and practice Yoga along with the instructor. With the books I had purchased open by my side, I began to experiment with other postures not on the tape. It took a few more visits to Kripalu, taking classes, until I felt comfortable with a sequence of postures, in Sanskrit called *asanas*, and breathing exercises, called *pranayamas*, I could do on my own every morning without playing the tape. From time to time, when my energy was low and I couldn't get to my Yoga mat on my own, I still used a tape to motivate me to practice. A few months passed, and I really did begin to feel better. I still had bad days when it was hard to get out of bed, but now the good days outweighed the bad ones.

After nine months of practicing every day and two or three more visits to Kripalu as a guest, I was driving in my van, listening to a Jean Houston tape that a friend who had attended her workshop had given me. Jean Houston is a well-known psychologist and healer. On the tape, Jean led the participants through a guided visualization, at the end of which they were to name themselves. I was probably a danger to myself and others that day as I entered an eyes-open kind of trance state while driving my car, and I would caution you not to do what I did. I was at a red light with my eyes half closed when Jean asked me to name myself. The light was still red, so I closed my eyes for an instant and was immediately filled with abundance, the feeling of abundance, the word *abundance,* and the name. As the light turned green, I accelerated, named myself Abundance, and laughed out loud. In that moment, my pockets were full!

Several days later, I was again sitting in my psychiatrist's office. I told her about the experience I'd had while listening to Jean Houston, and asked her if she didn't think it was time to try my life without antidepressants. She flipped her hand, as if my experience of abundance was transient, which of course it was, and as if to say I would not be able to maintain any semblance of happiness without my medication. She refused to discuss lowering my dosage. I continued to see her for a few more months. After all, we had been doing therapy for several years, and I loved her. Despite her habit of making blanket statements, there was love in the room, which I have come to believe is the essential element for change.

But more and more, I was seeing that her perception of me no longer matched the way I was seeing myself. Eventually, I realized that to manifest on the outside the abundant being I was on the inside, I would have to find a therapist who mirrored *my* view of myself, not hers. I went to a friend's psychiatrist, and after meeting with me over a period of weeks, he agreed that I was no longer a candidate for antidepressants. I did not go cold turkey but withdrew from the medication over a period of several weeks. That was in 1989, and I have not had need of medication since.

Aside from my biochemistry and a genetic predisposition to depression, there were reasons, carried from my own childhood, why for much of my life I had such a shaky sense of my own worth as a human being. The Yoga worked, not only to balance the biochemistry of my brain, to stimulate the endocrine system, and to create a state of healing relaxation, but also to dissolve those reasons why I believed I was unworthy of even my own love. I haven't forgotten the losses of my childhood, but I no longer carry them. And I don't need to tell myself those stories any longer.

As a reader, you may be saying to yourself something like "Yes, but she has a daily practice and she *teaches* Yoga." Take heart. After that very first Yoga class at Kripalu Center in 1989, I felt better. The immediate feel-good response encouraged me to practice often. I hope you will be encouraged by the news that within a year of beginning my Yoga practice, I was free of antidepressant medication.

I am a Yoga teacher who has recovered from depression through my practice of Yoga. In gratitude for my recovery, I am passionate about sharing the gifts I have received on my Yoga mat with others who suffer. Since my healing journey began in 1989 and through the research and writing of this book, I have been blessed by the guidance of many excellent teachers, psychotherapists, and *Jnana* Yogis (those who seek union through the study of sacred texts). As a Yoga teacher, I'm accustomed to leading others through the flow of breathing exercises and Yoga postures that invite each practitioner to come home to her natural state, that place where there are no separations, to reunite with the ground of her being. I invite you to let me lead you through the research, the stories, and the practices in this book, as though you were in my class, using what serves you and letting go of the rest. As I tell my students, "We are not creating a synchronized Yoga team. You are forming a new and healthier relationship with your body and mind. You have total permission to make this practice uniquely yours."

What's Wrong with the Medical Model?

This book does not advocate tossing your antidepressants in the trash. But when we broaden the view from our own experience to include the rising statistics on depression and the growing number of suicides, especially among young people, when we open our eyes to see how gravely the "empty pocket" syndrome is affecting so many of us, it is clear that antidepressants aren't the answer for the entire culture. They aren't even the real answer for the individual. We're treating the symptoms when we take our Paxil or our Celexa, but we're not addressing the root of our suffering; we do not meet our suffering at its source. Biomedicine treats symptoms. It treats the tumor, the virus, the infection, but it doesn't treat the whole person. It may even cure the disease, but it does not heal. It does not make whole what has been severed—our egos from the knowledge of our wholeness. In fact, some mental health professionals feel that medication can sometimes mask the core issues underlying the depression. As clinical psychologist and senior Yoga teacher Richard Miller says, "We cannot simply address the chemical component of depression and expect that depression will be alleviated."

Talk therapy, though a vital component in our individual recovery from depression and other psychological disturbances, also has its limits. If, as most psychologists agree, the seeds for our depression are sewn in infancy through patterns of relationships with significant others, *prior* to the acquisition of language, how can we root out the depression solely *through* language? Recovery from depression must include the body. Research shows that when we suffer trauma, it is mostly the lower, more primitive parts of the brain that are involved. According to Maryanna Eckberg, a psychologist who treats survivors of abuse, "A body-oriented treatment model speaks the language of these areas of the brain—sensation, perceptual experience and somatic responses. Cognitive restructuring is, of course, important, but the healing process must also include bodily experience."[2] Your own road to recovery from depression may be finding the balance of medication, talk therapy, and Yoga that works for you.

When my psychiatrist told me that I would always be "one of those people," she was alluding to the fact that I wasn't alone in my suffering. In fact, I was in good company. "The extent of inner feelings of emptiness and unworthiness in the Western psyche has seemed all but unbelievable to teachers raised in the East," says Buddhist psychoanalyst Mark Epstein.[3] In his book on psychotherapy from a Buddhist perspective, *Thoughts Without a Thinker*, Epstein talks about the human condition and the search for self. "We are aware of vague and disturbing feelings of emptiness, inauthenticity and alienation."[4] Most of us resist these vague feelings. Some of us work too hard or play too hard, giving rise to all manner of addictions that we hope will keep us from feeling our pain. We suffer and struggle and feel depressed, living behind a mask that psychologists call the "false self," avoiding the reality of who we really are.

"Living in this mortal body," said the Buddha, "is like living in a house on fire." We suffer. We have always suffered. So why do we see statistics for depression tripling in the years since World War II? Even before the tragic attack on the World Trade Center and the resulting increase in anxiety and depression all over the globe, depression was costing Americans big bucks. The biomedical Western model of treating depression is costing us more than 50 billion dollars a year. A University of Texas study released in 2001 says that bipolar disorder alone costs this country $24 billion a year, or between nearly $12,000 and $625,000 per patient per year, depending on the number of episodes.

Not only is depression costly, it kills. A five-year study conducted by the World Health Organization cites suicide from depression as the fourth-leading cause of death worldwide, and by 2020 it's expected to be the second, despite the increased availability of generic selective serotonin-reuptake inhibitors (SSRIs). When Eli Lilly introduced Prozac, the first SSRI, in 1987, it was going to revolutionize the treatment of depression. Millions of people worldwide take this antidepressant medication or one of the newer SSRIs, yet the number of suicides continues to mount. A Nottingham Medical School (UK) study released in 2001 has found that suicide is the leading cause of death among pregnant women and women with a child under one year old. According to a recent report published by the University of Washington's Kids Count, mental health problems have now surpassed injuries as the single most common reason for hospitalizations among children five to nineteen in the state of Washington. And currently, nationwide, suicide is the third-biggest killer of young people between the ages of fifteen and twenty-four.[5]

Something is terribly wrong with this picture. Why are so many of us serotonin deficient?

Research with rhesus monkeys has clearly demonstrated that major life stressors, such as early-childhood trauma, actually change brain chemistry. When baby monkeys were taken away from their mothers, their serotonin levels dropped.[6] Many other studies have shown that stress affects the levels of neurotransmitters like serotonin and dopamine. Could it be that the stressors inherent in our modern culture are the source of an international serotonin deficiency, causing depression in epidemic proportions? That the species mind of our postmodern world is depressed?

There may be good reason for this—the flip side of our ever-advancing technological culture. From the beginning of the Christian era, it took 1,500 years for our collective knowledge of the universe to double. Currently, scientists estimate that our collective knowledge doubles every eighteen months. But with that increased information has come a loss of connection, a loss of meaning, a loss of transcendence, the kind so easily achieved in ancient and indigenous cultures. Some of us carry that loss of meaning in the form of psychiatric symptoms. Many of us carry that loss of meaning in the form of depression. We are suffering in epidemic proportions—as individuals, as a community, and as a culture. We may have more information, but we have lost the truth of who we really are, the knowledge that at the core of our beings we are not separate from others and from the universe. The ancient Sanskrit texts call this forgetfulness *avidya*—ignorance. It is avidya that blinds us to our perfection, to the knowledge that we are born divine. There is no original sin in the system of Yoga. There is only wholeness and separation. When we forget that we belong to each other and to the universe, that we are deeply connected to all living beings, we feel separate and alone. And we suffer. Through the practice of Yoga, we awaken to the knowledge that what is most true about us, our soul, is always here—that, indeed, there is only one soul, whether we are in this human form in this lifetime or not. There is only one consciousness. The Yogis call this *Atman*. This is our true nature. When we remember this, our suffering disappears.

The Science of Positive Mental Health

You may be reading this book because you or someone you love is suffering the torment of depression. If you are considering the beginning of a Yoga practice as a means to lessen your anguish and change yourself in some way, you are on the right track. A daily Yoga practice will bring your physical body and your emotional body into balance, restoring a sense of well-being and energy. You will feel more energy, love yourself more, and have a happier life. Even beneath the chaos of mania, the agony of depression, Yoga says, you are whole; or as Yogi, psychotherapist, and author Stephen Cope puts it, "We are vaguely aware that, at least in some parallel universe, we are unutterably fine just the way we are."[7]

When you step onto your Yoga mat, you are reminded of that wholeness, and the practice clears a pathway through your symptoms to the ground of your being, that which is your natural state. "Depression," says Richard Miller, "is the feeling of separation from self." The underlying Yogic approach to treating depression is "informed by the knowledge that there is no separation." The teacher "stands firm in the truth of oneness." In other words, Yoga begins with the question What is *right* with me? Not What is wrong with me?

Here in the West, we are accustomed to thinking of mental health from the perspective of illness—how best to understand and treat our symptoms. But we practice Yoga as preventative and positive medicine. Just as the immune system is strengthened against the common cold and other viruses with daily practice, the emotional body is strengthened as well. The highs, the lows, the extremes of all the emotions are brought into balance by the physical practice, and the mind is soothed by the philosophy. In every stage of Yoga, you will find relief from obsessive negative thinking. When you are first learning a pose and moving into it, you cannot possibly obsess about what you should have said in the meeting this morning. To learn the pose, your mind must focus on the details of alignment. Later, when you're in the pose and you allow your mind to become absorbed in the sensations in your body, you are very far from your everyday troubles.

It must be said that the ancient Yogis who developed and practiced Yoga did *not* do so with the goal of recovering from depression, or even of maintaining positive mental health. Their goal was liberation (*moksha*), the total freedom from suffering, and positive mental health was a side effect of that goal. But we are a more psychological culture, and for good reason: While Indian children more often grow up with a sense of community and connectedness, often riding on mother's hip until they are old enough to walk and living in extended families, our childhoods are more often fragmented, more about separation than connectedness. As a culture, we look to Yogic techniques as a way to heal that separation. For me and for most of my students practicing Yoga in the West today, the goal is simply to maintain physical and emotional well-being. For us, perhaps moksha will be the side effect of our goal of maintaining, through Yogic techniques, positive mental health.

Two Yoga Strategies for Depression

Willful Practice

There are numerous ways that Yoga can help alleviate depression, but there are two different approaches to dealing with the feelings of depression. The first approach addresses the symptoms of depression by advocating a practice that keeps introspection to a minimum. For example, B.K.S. Iyengar suggests that people who suffer from depression practice with their eyes open and avoid holding forward bends or practicing Corpse Pose, known in Sanskrit as *Shavasana*. He and the teachers he has trained recommend some very specific postures (asanas) for symptom relief. One of the world's leading Iyengar teachers, Patricia Walden, who has done extensive exploration of Yoga poses that help her students in their recovery from depression, offers specific suggestions, some of which we will look at in Chapter Five. She says that when she first met Mr. Iyengar in the 1960s in Cambridge, Massachusetts, he told her she would never get depressed if she kept her armpits open. This may be good advice for some, especially those suffering from seasonal affective disorder (SAD), whose source of depression is the weather and lack of sunlight. As we'll explore more thoroughly later in the book, the emphasis in Iyengar Yoga is on willful practices (*tapas*) that keep the mind from brooding.

Self-Study

But for many of us who are grieving or who suffer from the more common low-grade depression known as *dysthymia*, I prefer the second strategy for dealing with depression—"the only way out is through" approach. In the tradition in which I've received my primary training, Kripalu Yoga, the mat itself becomes the place you show up with your whole self—your angry self if you're angry, your grieving self if you're grieving. The emphasis of this approach is on self-observation (*svadhyaya*). This is no ordinary analysis, but rather a recognition and an acceptance of the way things are. I acknowledge that today I have sad feelings, but I also see that I am not my sad feelings, that I have a self that is bigger than these fleeting emotions.

This is especially true when we practice long holdings of postures in order to witness, with equanimity and awareness, all of our feelings, without reaction. Holding gives us an opportunity to notice the places in the body where energy is blocked, where emotion or even trauma is stored. These energy blocks, known in Sanskrit as *samskaras,* show up as strong sensation or numbness, and they restrict the free flow of energy through the body. On an emotional level, they may be responsible for restricting the open expression of our feelings. Eventually these energy blocks can lead to symptoms and then illness, both physical and mental. By focusing the breath and the awareness, where the sensation is strongest, we allow energy to begin to flow in that area of the body. On a physical level, as we hold we create a pressure gradient in the contraction of the muscles involved in the posture, so that in addition to the emotional clearing that can take place upon release, there is a physical cleansing of the lymphatic system. The practice itself brings the emotional body back into balance. In Chapter Three, we'll find out how this happens when we look at the research that establishes these physiological and psychological benefits, but first let's look at a bit of basic Yoga philosophy to understand the Yogic view of our suffering.

The Yoga Tree

There is archaeological evidence that Yoga postures were practiced thousands of years ago in the pre-Columbian cultures of the Americas. In India, the secrets of Yoga were not written down, but passed from master to student for thousands of years, until Patanjali compiled *The Yoga Sutras* around 200 C.E. The *Sutras* are the foundation of our current understanding of Classical Yoga. A few hundred years later, several other important Yoga books, like the *Hatha Yoga Pradipika*, recorded the specific practices of Hatha Yoga. It is from these ancient texts that our modern Yoga system has developed.

Yoga is a systematic method for maintaining optimum physical and emotional health. That method is called the Eight-Limbed Path, and it includes postures (asanas), breathing exercises (pranayamas), concentration, and meditation. It even includes a system of values, which we will discuss in Chapter Four. The method also recommends a way of working with our negative mind states that, much like cognitive therapy, helps us break through our self-limiting beliefs.

In some traditions the student progresses sequentially through the Eight-Limbed Path of the Classical Hatha Yoga system. In other words, he learns only the postures at first, preparing the body to receive the breath. In such a tradition, when your teacher feels you are ready, she might teach you some simple breathing exercises (pranayamas). Only after a time of practicing postures (asanas) and more advanced breathing exercises (pranayamas) would you be deemed ready to meditate. First, you would learn techniques to withdraw your senses from the world around you so that your focus remains inside. Then you would learn concentration techniques that help to clear and focus your mind. Finally, you would learn to meditate. Ultimately, your meditation will bring you to a healing state, a blissful feeling wherein you may lose the sense of yourself as a being separate from the universe and gain a momentary sense of union.

As someone who has suffered from depression and has worked with many depressed students, I feel that this wonderful system of healing can and should be practiced not one by one, like steps on a ladder, but rather like a newly planted sapling that grows branches in all directions. To overcome your depression, it's important that you work with your breath from the very beginning. You may not feel comfortable meditating until you have released tension from your body and strengthened your spine to enable you to sit. And you may want to work with your breath and with the Yogic practice of affirmations in order to slow the spiral of negative thoughts before you meditate. However, if you are depressed, it's important that you accompany the physical practice of the postures with your growing knowledge and experience of the breath from the moment you first step onto your Yoga mat. In the chapters that follow, we will talk about each branch of your Yoga tree and how you can root yourself in positive mental health.

Yoga Asks: Why Suffer?

The classical Yoga scriptures tell us that we suffer because we are bound too tightly to current reality by the five afflictions (*kleshas*). As we've seen, the first and foremost bind is ignorance (*avidya*). As we live farther and farther from the truth of our wholeness, we become ignorant of that wholeness and live as though we are separate and alone. We forget our magnificence because of the other four afflictions that arise out of avidya. Because of our own "I-ness" (*asmita*) we identify too much with this body, this mind, these emotions. Out of this identification the third and fourth afflictions arise—attraction (*raga*) and aversion (*dvesha*). We define ourselves by what we love and what we hate, and cling to life. Our fear of change, and particularly the final change, death, is the fifth affliction (*abhinivesha*).[8]

The ancient Yogis believed that through the practice of Yoga, we are given an opportunity to wake up from our ignorance, to transcend our identification with our bodies, our clinging to what we love, our avoidance of what we hate, our fear of death. Each time we step on the Yoga mat, we are given the opportunity to remember who we really are. This continues to be verified for me through my own experience. I have seen my life change in remarkable ways over the fifteen years that I've maintained a daily practice of Yoga. I have suffered in those fifteen years in response to events and losses in my life, but I have not fallen into a depression again in all that time. Through my practice, I am constantly reminded that I am not my body, not my emotions, not my job as a Yoga teacher, my job as a writer, not my house, not my desires, not my failures, not even my thoughts, and I'm certainly not "one of those people who will always have empty pockets." I love my job, I love my house, I love my daughter and my beloved, but I am not any of these. Every day, my practice lets me touch my natural state, that universal place in myself, what the Buddhists might call "emptiness" or "no self," what the Yogis might call "*Atman*," or "Self" with a capital *S*. "Emptiness" or "wholeness," "Self" or "no self," or even "abundance"—by any name, my experience of this state is one of healing and peace so profound that I have not suffered from depression since 1989.

Getting Started

Most of us come to Yoga practice after years of abuse to our bodies— exercising without stretching, or no exercise, overeating, or addictions to substances, sex, or work. Our bodies are stiff in places, and we may have weakness in certain organs. If we are depressed, our energy is probably low and we may bring to the mat a mind troubled by negative self-talk, worry, and fear. If you are in a state of struggle in your daily life, it is best to start simply with a routine of gentle warm-ups, followed by a simple Yoga sequence of stretches in which you invite your mind to pay attention to the sensations in your body, maintaining a calm and steady breath as you practice. Your routine will likely include side stretching, forward-bending poses that stretch the muscles in your back and develop a strong and flexible spine, backward-bending poses that open the chest, and twisting postures that massage the internal organs and loosen the hips. Even with a basic beginning routine, you will feel the effects immediately.

Many people who suffer from depression don't even know they are depressed. But if you are reading this book and perhaps even practicing Yoga, you've already begun to access your own healing power. Though you may be suffering now, you will find that your mind is a wellspring of mental health, your body has the potential to stretch and change beyond the limits of your preconceived notions, and your capacity to love yourself and others is growing.

If you aren't currently practicing Yoga, find a class, learn a practice, then commit to it. Most likely, you bathe your body and brush your teeth every day. Think of your practice as an essential part of your hygiene and it will become so. I would no more start my day without Yoga than I would get up and go to work without brushing my teeth. Actually, there are rare occasions when, because of travel, I don't practice in the morning, and I usually feel slightly less centered than I would like. Once you've begun a class with a qualified teacher, commit to practicing every day on your own, even if it's for only ten minutes. Simple spinal flexes on your hands and knees, a twist, a mountain pose, remembering to breathe long and deep through your nostrils, may be a good beginning.

When you willfully bring yourself to the Yoga mat, especially on days when you feel overwhelmed by inertia, you will feel marvelous after your practice. Developing this habit of showing up on your mat, "stepping up to the plate," even when you're feeling some resistance, makes you feel very good about yourself. The effect of gently using your will has a ripple effect in your daily life. How often do we procrastinate, putting off what we know we must do—paying the bills, making the difficult phone call, writing the proposal—often using our depression as the excuse? But how good it feels when we actually begin the dreaded project, and how much better we feel when it's done! Coming to your mat every day cultivates an attitude of saying "yes" to yourself and the work you must do.

Just yesterday, I had a direct experience of stepping through my resistance. I received a letter from the editor of this book, suggesting major structural revisions and a somewhat different approach to the material. Of course, I wanted her to love the manuscript just as it was, so two nights ago, when I first read her letter, my own negative self-talk kicked in: *I can't do it! I'll never be able to finish on time!* But her letter was well-reasoned and persuasive, and after a good night's sleep and morning Yoga practice, I read it again and recognized that not only would her suggestions make this a better book, but that I *could* do it, and in fact, couldn't wait to get started! I could have taken to my bed for a day with a blanket over my head, as one author friend does when she hears from her editor. Instead, I dove in right after my morning Yoga practice, forgoing e-mails and my workout in the weight room. The day of writing was one of the most enjoyable I've had. I felt glorious afterward.

"There's nothing more satisfying than to acknowledge to yourself that you are working though your own resistance," says senior Iyengar

Yoga instructor Patricia Walden. "Practicing at these times of inertia builds strength of character, confidence, self-esteem, willpower. You are building *tapas* (inner fire)." As your practice becomes stronger, you become stronger. And you take that strength off the mat and into your daily life. With each session on your mat, you are building the strength to break through old patterns and past conditioning.

"But what if I have no self-discipline?" you might ask. "What if rolling out my mat requires more commitment than I can muster?" Just try it. Yoga feels so good that you will want to return to your mat. The self-discipline evolves out of your practice, not the other way around. You will roll out your mat tomorrow morning not because you are committed to improving yourself in some way, but simply because it feels good to stretch your body, and because you feel so much better afterward. You'll notice a difference in your energy level and your outlook all day. So the next morning, you'll want to practice again. As the twelve-step recovery programs advocate, "take it one day at a time." And little by little, you will begin to change. The self-discipline you are evolving on your mat will flow into your daily life.

You may even find that difficult choices, like giving up an addictive behavior, become a little easier. Many Yogis report that their addictions and bad choices simply fall away in the heat and discipline of their practice. It was easy for me, for example, to give up eating red meat, as I simply lost the desire for it. This is not to say that Yoga eliminates addictive cravings for alcohol, food, drugs, or sex. But a daily Yoga practice has helped many practitioners manage their addictions and their obsessions. There are still times when I am riding my bike that I catch myself thinking the same thoughts again and again. What I will say to my friend, what he will say to me, what I should have said, and on and on and on. This never happens when I am on my Yoga mat, whether doing my own practice or leading others. And though I can still find myself fretting too much, making, as my grandmother might say, a mountain out of a molehill, my practice has helped me develop an awareness of this pattern. I can usually catch myself, breathe deeply, acknowledge my clinging thoughts, then let them go.

But wait, here I am talking about practicing every day, even when you don't feel like it, and you may not have even begun. The last thing I want to do is overwhelm you or create even more anxiety about how you will fit a daily Yoga session into your already crowded day. Now, this may sound like a contradiction, but *don't worry about it.* If you find the right class, start there. Take a baby step. You will feel so good afterward that you'll want to take a bigger step. I am passionate about sharing the knowledge I've gained through my own experience of Yoga, not only because of my recovery from depression but because it's a treatment you and I can do for ourselves. Once you've learned a basic routine, you can self-medicate every day, and unlike drugs or alcohol, your practice will strengthen and purify your body and mind. It is powerful to become your own healer!

But you and I both know that when you are feeling depressed, there are times when doing something that's good for you, even if you know you'll feel better afterward, is the last thing you're able to do. Depression creates its own inertia, and it's hard to break that. The lethargy can be so strong that you cannot even get out of bed. What to do? Take a small step, even if it's imperceptible to anyone around you. Your first small step may simply be that you sit up in bed instead of lying down. Your next small step may be inhaling deeply through your nostrils, holding the breath for a moment, then exhaling. Maybe you'll do that five times, maybe twenty. Notice how you feel. You might just have mustered enough energy to climb out of bed.

Once you're out of bed, your Yoga practice may simply be going outside to breathe deeply, practicing some of the breathing exercises described in Chapter Six, or taking a walk in which you watch your breath or count your steps. Most practitioners find that when they do one small thing, like a pranayama breathing exercise, they then have the energy to do the next small thing, until they are soon moving through a practice.

Finding a Teacher

Okay, so you're out of bed, you've turned off the TV, you've walked past the refrigerator and the cabinet where all those carbohydrates are stored. You have decided that today, for a change, you will not numb out. And if you are reading this book and you're not already practicing Yoga, you're ready to find a class. Chances are, you live in a place where there are several styles of Yoga from which to choose. Ask your friends, or the woman at the gym who stretches between rounds on the Cybex machines. Someone among your circle of friends and family is already practicing Yoga and loving it. Ask several people about their teachers. Do they feel inspired and empowered to stretch a little deeper? Do they feel safe? When the class is over, do they feel like hugging someone? Are they grateful? Yes, there may be a style of Yoga practice that suits your constitution more than another, and eventually you will gravitate to studying that practice. We'll talk about the various styles of practice more in Chapter Five. But for now, even more important than determining the most appropriate style of practice is finding the right teacher for you to begin. Does she understand the basics of body mechanics so that your informant feels safe in the class? Does he move slowly through the basics of properly aligning the spine? And most important, in my opinion, does she encourage you to accept your body, with all its current limitations, just as it is? Acceptance is at the heart of Yoga. It is the first step toward change. It's like the importance of locating yourself on the map before you can plan the route toward your destination. Does your potential new Yoga teacher encourage you to believe that all the tools you need to reach your destination are already inside you? If something in his attitude makes you feel that he owns the tools and will lend them to you only while you stand in a pose in his class, then you probably want to look elsewhere. And if, while practicing, the Yoga teacher says something that makes you feel ashamed of your body in or out of the pose, again, you should probably move on to another teacher.

A magnificent eighty-three-year-old Yoga teacher, who in 1977 was one of the first program directors for the Kripalu Yoga teacher training, said in her gentle class just the other day, "You can never do anything wrong in a Yoga class, just different." I wouldn't go that far. Certainly, you can injure yourself in Yoga, usually by stretching too deeply into a pose before your body is properly warmed up, but the sentiment is correct. And the context for her comment was a lovely class of slow, gentle stretching with lots of warm-ups. There was little a student could have done in that class that would have caused him harm. Going to a class is not about accomplishing the perfect posture. It's about learning to build a new relationship with your body. It's about learning a practice that will strengthen and purify your body and mind. It's about your recovery from depression. And for that you need a safe and nurturing container. If you're ready to begin a practice and are looking for a teacher right now, skip ahead to Chapter Five, which may help you decide what you need in a class and a teacher. But please come back here, because there's so much more I want to share with you that will help make your first exploration of Yoga a healing journey.

The Body of the Book

Let's begin the journey with an overview. Thousands of years of Yogic wisdom and experience have given rise to a science of positive mental health that is deeply rooted in the fertile ground of Yogic philosophy. In this book, we'll explore the ways in which Yoga philosophy and practice, including postures, breath work, and meditation, can help you manage or even overcome your depression.

Chapter Two lays the groundwork for a better understanding of your own depression and for how Yoga, as a complete system, can address your needs. You will find stories of Yoga practitioners who suffered from various kinds of depression—dysthymia or chronic low-level depression, major depression, anxiety-based depression, and bipolar disorder. From these stories, you may begin to identify your own unique symptoms and begin to see how you, like the practitioners in these stories, can overcome them.

Chapter Three is for the scientific-minded among us. Medical science is coming closer to establishing the empirical evidence to support practitioners' claims that the practice of Yoga, including breathing exercises (*pranayamas*) and meditation, has beneficial effects on our emotional well-being, our mental acuity, and in many cases, the alleviation of our depression. In this chapter we'll look at some of the research that gives us an idea of how Yoga works to heal us and why.

Chapter Four outlines the basic philosophical principles of Yoga, including the Yoga system of values, so that from a Yogic perspective, you understand why your practice is changing your life off the mat.

Chapter Five looks at several theories of asana posture practice and takes you through a very personal journey—my own moment-to-moment experience on my Yoga mat.

Chapter Six will explore the pranayama breathing practices that calm the anxious mind, and we'll talk about breathing practices that stimulate the mind dulled by depression.

Chapter Seven looks at the healing experiences people have had when they practice Sudharshan Kriya, a technique that is especially effective for depression.

In Chapter Eight, we'll look at various meditation techniques that have brought solace to practitioners suffering from depression, so that you can begin to consider the kind of practice that is right for you.

In Chapter Nine, we'll dive deeper into the most authentic expression of Yoga—not the doing, but the undoing, the releasing of the obstacles to your freedom, so that you can see your own potential for creative self-expression. Here, you'll read about the ways in which the long holding of Yoga postures can, with guidance, release the traumas and losses we carry in our bodies.

In the final chapter, we'll talk about other aspects of the Yoga system—community, devotion, and service—that can help you move the focus of your attention out beyond your own self-limiting pain.

And in the appendix, you'll find many resources—Web sites, books, videotapes, and programs—to help you deepen your knowledge of Yoga and to find places to practice where you live.

Throughout the book I will, through the generosity of my students and colleagues, share stories about people's lives that will enable you to recognize the common ground of suffering you have with them and will, I hope, inspire you to begin or strengthen your own daily practice of Yoga. All of the stories in this book are true, but most of them are not factual. Often names have been changed, identities disguised, and composites have been drawn. In the fictionalizing of the many stories I have heard and experienced firsthand, I seek only to explore the emotional truth of the narrative. As you read about others who have recovered from depression, I hope that the moments of self-recognition brighten the light through the window of your suffering.

A Word About Practice

At the end of each chapter, I will offer you a Yoga Experience. These are simple Yogic tools to help you soothe yourself if you're feeling anxious and other tools to energize yourself if you are feeling depressed. However, this book is not meant to be a guide to developing your own practice. There are excellent books and videotapes on the market that take you, step by step, through a beginning Yoga routine, and many of them are listed in the Resources. It is far better, however, to begin with a teacher. The breathing exercises, postures, visualizations, relaxations, and affirmations I suggest come from various Yoga traditions. Taken together, these Yoga Experiences are not a complete sequence, but they can be woven into your home practice, along with the routine you have learned from your teacher. Though they are simple enough to try at home, they are not meant to be a substitute for learning Yoga from a qualified teacher who can help you adapt and modify a Yoga routine to your own needs.

These are techniques that my teachers, my colleagues, my students, and I have used to help balance the emotional body. Yogis have used many of these practices for thousands of years, whereas some techniques are new developments based on my own research and experimentation. In the spirit of *svadhyaya*—self-reflection and observation—I invite you to experiment and explore as you read this book and work with a Yoga teacher, developing a routine that is your own route to positive mental health.

Remembering

Let's return to my therapist's couch in Providence, Rhode Island, twenty years ago. "Empty pockets," she said. I felt she was dooming me to an unsatisfying life in which no matter how much I loved and was loved, no matter what I achieved, I would always yearn for more. Today I understand that sometimes my pockets feel full to overflowing, that I have abundant energy, abundant love, and a solid sense of self that is rooted in the knowledge of my wholeness, my feeling that I am not separate from the universe. When I forget who I am, I have only to return to my Yoga mat to remember. But I also understand that though those pockets are chock full of blessings, from time to time they can still feel empty. It is my embrace of that emptiness that brings me closest to the truth of being human. I would never wish for a life without pain. Pain is my teacher; it is what allows me to feel the suffering of others. I rejoice that I have a heart big enough to break over and over again. And because I can accept the emptiness I sometimes feel, I have learned that it is *in my yearning* that I am most fulfilled. The thirteenth-century mystic and poet Rumi said, "When you look for God, God is in the look in your eyes." Empty pockets are our reality, the source of both our suffering and our wholeness.

yoga experience

Many suggestions for specific practices will be offered throughout the book, but for you to choose which practices will be most effective for you, it's important for you to think about your depression, to understand the nature of your state of mind. You want to learn to meet your depression or your anxiety with your practice and move the energy in a healing direction. We will explore the various states of a depressed mind in more depth in the next chapter. For now, you will simply be observing your energy. If you find that you have too much energy, as in anxiety or mania, you may feel more comfortable beginning with a more active practice that matches your state of mind. Then gradually, over the course of your session, you will begin to slow your practice down until you are using soothing, calming postures and breathing exercises and are finally able to fully relax. On the other hand, if your depression is characterized by a lack of energy, you may feel more comfortable if you begin with a breath that closely follows your own, perhaps shallow, breath. Then gradually, over the course of your session, you may begin to introduce a more active breath with more expansive movement, moving slowly toward an energizing practice that awakens your life force, or *prana*.

Meditation

Let's begin with a simple meditation practice that allows you to calmly observe your state of mind so that you can determine how to begin your practice. Sit in a comfortable position in a chair or on the floor. If you choose to sit on the floor, you can sit off the edge of a cushion, with your legs crossed in Easy Pose, so your spine is elevated and your knees are lower than your hips. You can also use cushions under your knees and padding beneath your ankles. It's important that you find a position where you can sit without discomfort and with your spine erect for five minutes or so.

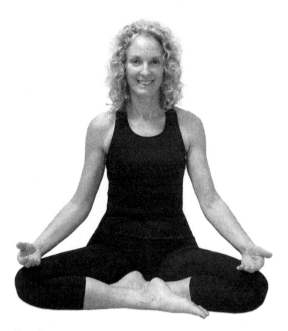

Easy Pose

Begin by noticing the breath as it moves in and out through the tips of your nostrils. Notice the temperature of the breath. Can you distinguish which nostril is dominant? Is your breath rough or smooth? Notice whether the inhalation is longer than the exhalation, or if the exhalation is longer than the inhalation. Just observe, without judgment, how you are breathing right now.

If your normal breath is, for example, three counts in and four counts out, observe it for several breaths, then see if you can extend the length of both the inhalation and the exhalation. For instance, you might try four counts in and six counts out. Do this for several breaths.

Then follow the thread of your breath through your body, noticing what sensations are present without any judgment about them. You are cultivating the witness of your own experience. Can you be at ease with the sensations you are feeling in your physical body? Can you observe without reacting?

Next, follow the thread of your breath through your emotional body, noticing what feelings are present without any judgment about them. Just acknowledge the emotion, or lack of emotion, numbness perhaps, and trust that your practice will bring balance into your emotional body.

Next, dive beneath your physical and emotional body, beneath your unique manifestations of self, home to the ground of your being, that place of witness to all that you are thinking and feeling, that place that knows no boundaries, no separation. And from this place of wholeness, of witness, begin to notice where the feeling or lack of feeling that you have identified is stored in your body. Do you feel a heaviness (or flightiness) in your chest? Your belly? Your head? Does the feeling have a color? A weight? A texture? You are the witness of your feelings, observing them with awareness and equanimity, the two pillars of Yogic practice. Receive the numbness or the flightiness as if you were welcoming a friend. Let the feeling know that here, on your cushion and on your Yoga mat, it will not be shoved aside or stuffed. Tell the feeling or its lack that in this place even numbness, even anxiety will be embraced with acceptance and compassion.

Now invite any benevolent energies you wish into this place, perhaps someone in your life who has said "yes" to you, or a deity or higher power that gives you strength. Sit for as long as you like with this energy.

From this place of wholeness and compassion for yourself, ask what you need for your practice today. What kind of practice would suit you? Do you need to begin slowly, meeting the heaviness where it is and then gradually becoming more active with an energizing practice? Or do you need to begin more actively, meeting the anxious feeling and then gradually slowing down into a soothing, calming practice? See if you can answer this question from this place of wholeness.

When you're ready to return, imagine that you are looking down on your physical body from high above. Look with compassion at this body that has carried you through all the years of this lifetime, through sadness and joy, abundance and emptiness, achievement and loss. Begin to breathe more deeply, until you are comfortable opening your eyes and beginning your practice.

a house on fire —
the ways we suffer

I tell you, deep inside you is a fountain of bliss, a fountain of joy.
Deep inside your center core is truth, light, love, there is no guilt there,
there is no fear there. Psychologists have never looked deep enough.

—SRI SRI RAVI SHANKAR, Art of Living Foundation Founder[1]

In the early nineties, I was often on staff for self-discovery programs at
Kripalu Center. I remember assisting psychologist Rasmani Deborah Orth as she led an exercise that culminated in a sharing. People were
sitting on their cushions in small groups, taking turns describing their
experiences. As I wandered from group to group, offering tissues, I
noticed that whoever was sharing was tearfully telling her group about a
difficult time in her life. I heard bits and pieces of stories about sexual
assault, emotional neglect, physical abuse. I watched as listeners' eyes

softened and filled with empathy and their bodies leaned toward the person who was sharing. I could almost feel my own capacity for love and compassion expanding with the speaker's sad story. In my sadness, I felt connected to the speaker and her pain, and that made me feel more alive. Writer and Yogi Anne Cushman, former editor of *Yoga Journal,* puts it this way: "Our grief shows us how we are 'attached.' But it also shows us the glorious part of our attachment—that we are woven into the fabric of the world, that we are linked to everything that is."[2]

As I moved around the room, listening to one painful story after another, I began to see before me what I had only held as an idea in my mind—that suffering is universal. No one is immune. Each story was different—some horrible, some mildly disturbing—but in the moment of its telling, the suffering of the speaker was the same. Near the end of the sharing, I stopped by a circle where a man was having difficulty describing, through his tears, how as a boy he'd been beaten and had his shoes stolen by two older boys on the way home from school. When he got home, his mother, rather than comforting him, became angry with him over the loss of the shoes and sent him to his room. Then I moved to another circle, where a woman sobbed in equal measure about how, as a child, she'd never been allowed to sing at the dining room table, something her best friend's parents encouraged. In their stories, two very different kinds of pain were expressed, and yet, in that moment, both the man and the woman knew suffering.

"Depression is the common cold of the deluded human being," says Stephen Cope. "And according to the Buddha, all human beings are quite deluded." Indeed, none of us can escape the pain of daily life. We lose pets, parents, children, beloved partners, best friends. Our friends betray us, our lovers abandon us, our stories are rejected, our ideas are mocked, our paintings are ignored. None of us is spared loss. We see the suffering of others less fortunate on the nightly news, hear their impassioned or terrified voices on the radio as we drive home from work. None of us grows old without grief. And grief is an important emotion, a cleansing emotion that comes as a natural response to loss. If we don't want to become sick, it's important to allow ourselves the experience of sad feelings when they arise. According to Alexander Lowen, M.D., the founder of bioenergetics, the suppression of feeling creates a predisposition toward depression. He says that a person suffering from depression is "like a swimmer with an anchor tied to his leg. No matter how hard he tries to swim to the surface, the anchor drags him down."[3]

Now let's consider the ways in which we humans are prone to suffer.

Grief

> Ah, woe is me! Winter is come and gone.
> But grief returns with the revolving year.
>
> —PERCY BYSSHE SHELLEY, *Adonis*

Sadness is like the flow of water. Our tears can cleanse us, emptying out old, held-in pain. On the other hand, when sadness continues too long, that watery flow of cleansing emotion can harden like ice into depression. The recent loss of a loved one is the most frequently reported catalyst for acute depression. But all losses, including traumatic events—both personal, like divorce, or national, like the effects of terrorism and war, or even natural events like earthquakes—can cause severe immediate or delayed depression, particularly among people who may have a genetic or biological predisposition. When grief becomes depression, our biochemistry changes; a biochemical madness descends upon the neurotransmitters of the brain. There is a reduction in the chemicals serotonin and norepinephrine and an increase in the stress hormone cortisol. New research indicates that the hippocampus, the part of the brain responsible for our ability to remember, may actually shrink.[4]

It's vitally important to feel our sadness and grief. If you are distracting yourself from your true feelings of sadness by working too much or eating too much or drinking too much or even practicing Yoga in some driven, goal-oriented way, you are only damming the flow. If you're lucky, the dam will eventually burst in a nurturing and safe environment. But if you're really good at distracting yourself, you may be able to freeze the emotion. The result: a depression, perhaps characterized by numbness. "Grief," says psychologist Rubin Naiman, "can be seen as a periodic, voluntary descent into what Jung calls negrido, the dark primal substrate of life. If we resist, the old scaly hand of depression comes up out of this swamp and involuntarily drags us down." Like many others, Naiman believes that most of our emotional distress arises from "faulty resolutions to loss—that is, bad grieving."

I've seen the effects of grief firsthand in many of my classes. John DeCoville, a fifty-five-year-old computer engineer, was grieving the loss of his wife when I met him. Ingrid had died of complications from a debilitating kidney disease three months earlier, and when John's sorrow failed to lessen, his hospice bereavement counselor suggested he try Yoga. He told me later that he'd wept in his car as he'd driven down to the class. The past week had been particularly hard, and that afternoon he'd picked up photographs of Ingrid that had lain undeveloped in his camera since her death. Still reeling from his losses, he felt as though he was descending again into what he calls "the pit of hell."

In class that evening, I began with a centering meditation, during which I invited the students to become aware of what they were experiencing in their emotional bodies, without judging or trying to change anything. I suggested that they watch, with compassion, all that arose for them during the practice, and to let the practice itself bring balance into the emotional body. During the opening breathing exercises, John's mood began to lift. "Without any mental processing," he says, "I was suddenly feeling better." During the warm-ups, I led a sequence that you'll find described in the Yoga Experience at the end of this chapter. "I was still feeling my feelings," John said, "but a complete sense of freedom came over me when we followed your instruction to 'Fly up' from the Child Pose." After that, he says he felt a sudden relief from intense pressure. "In the hours that followed I felt grateful to God, safe, loved."

Over the course of the next few days, John thanked me many times for what he called his "sudden turnaround," and said that he was better able to accept his grief without judgment. "I think that accepting my current state is a very important gate I must go through before I can experience new things. Not accepting has kept me stuck in a kind of hell." New to Yoga, John is continuing his practice as a way, along with counseling, to help him manage his grief.

Post-Traumatic Stress Disorder (PTSD)

Whenever suffering comes, I will find a form to meet it.

How can I not be there?

Pain will always open your eyes to see me.

—SUZANNE IRONBITER, "The Goddess's Promise"[5]

It is not the aim of this book to catalogue the many emotional states and psychiatric disturbances to which we humans are subject. However, depression often accompanies PTSD, and in the wake of rising acts of terror around the globe, I want to offer hope to those suffering from the consequences of traumatic events.

Shoshanna is a thirty-two-year-old epidemiologist who spent a year living in Israel during a time of intense conflict and strife. Her best friend was killed when a bomb exploded at a wedding that Shoshanna was also attending. Soon after that, she witnessed a bus exploding. She returned to the United States in an agitated state. In her nightmares, bodies exploded and children ran screaming down the street. She often awakened in tears from dreams where something important was lost. Whenever she heard a loud noise, she experienced frightening flashbacks to the terrible wedding scene. She was often shaky and unable to do her work. When she was diagnosed with PTSD, in addition to medication and therapy, she began a regular Yoga practice. "The focus on the details of the postures and on my breathing calms my mind," she says. "Whatever worries or fears or troubling thoughts I begin with dissolve as I practice. And I feel a lot better for hours afterward." Shoshanna hasn't had a nightmare in more than a year, and feels that though she'll carry the loss of her friend and the memory of that night for the rest of her life, it no longer devastates her to think about it. She maintains an almost daily Yoga practice and is no longer on medication.

PTSD may occur when a person is threatened with death or serious injury, or witnesses such a threat to others. Someone involved in such an event may respond with feelings of intense fear, helplessness, or horror. Afterward, she may develop the symptoms of PTSD, which include flashbacks, either through thoughts or nightmares, extreme efforts to avoid any activity or people that remind her of the event, or what psychologists call "heightened arousal." This last category of symptoms might include irritability, sleep disturbance, and irrational fears of being unsafe.

Psychiatrist Roy King has been on the faculty of the Department of Psychiatry and Behavioral Science at Stanford University since 1984 and is now an associate professor. In his private psychotherapy practice, when appropriate, King recommends that patients begin a Yoga practice by taking a class. He has found Yogic techniques, particularly pranayama breathing exercises and visualization, effective in treating PTSD and panic attacks.

One of Dr. King's patients experienced heightened arousal after she heard a report on child pornography on National Public Radio. As a child, the patient had been sexually molested, and when she heard the news story, she had a severe stress reaction that included an immediate sense of reliving the terror. According to Dr. King, she was "shaky, sweaty, tremulous." In their session the next day, Dr. King offered her a breathing technique and a visualization technique to block the visual flashbacks of her abuse. "Just learning how to breathe," says Dr. King, "can transform the nature of someone's thoughts about the trauma to which they were subjected."

Janis Carter, a psychiatrist in Brisbane, Australia, uses Iyengar-style Yoga therapy in her clinical practice with patients suffering from depression and PTSD. When her patients practice the Yoga she prescribes at home, she has found that they have a diminished need for medication. Even patients who believe themselves to be too inflexible to practice Yoga have benefited from their work with her. "I have had a patient do a backbend over a fitball [a plastic ball inflated to the size of a large beach ball], hold it for some time, and achieve a marked mood change within a session. The change in mood continued for two days, before it started to slip." For safety, she places the fitball against the wall, and the patient walks his hands down the wall. "There is no pharmacological agent that can cause such a quick response and maintain it for twenty-four hours," she says.

Janis Carter has just completed a six-week study with nine men suffering from PTSD. The men attended a once-a-week class where they were taught a sequence of postures designed by B.K.S. Iyengar to treat depression.[6] Though they were encouraged to practice at home, only a few of them did. On both the CESD self-rating scale for depression and the Hamilton Scale, rated by the psychiatrist, the men improved enormously. Out of the nine participants, all of whom in the first week were severely depressed, several showed no sign of depression by the third week, and none of them registered even mild depression in either measurement by the end of six weeks.

Peter Beard, a Vietnam veteran and retired mechanical engineer diagnosed with PTSD, began working with Dr. Carter in 2001. He served in South Vietnam as a crew commander and says he was "exposed to more than my share of carnage and futility." His experiences in Vietnam were "impossible to come to terms with. PTSD symptoms have had a serious grip on my life since returning from Vietnam in 1970." These symptoms seemed to worsen about five years ago, when Peter began to drink more heavily. His wife found his short temper, anxiety, and paranoia difficult to deal with. He experienced flashbacks and nightmares from which he would awaken in a sweat. His attention to detail was impaired, and he lost interest in most of the things that had given him relief. Mostly he wanted to be alone. As a result of his worsening PTSD, his marriage was threatened. When Peter went into treatment with Dr. Carter, he expected to be put on medication. Instead, she showed him basic postures and prescribed a daily practice. "In the eighteen months I've practiced Yoga for an average of forty minutes a day, I have managed to stabilize most of the PTSD symptoms. Yoga fits in well with my daily routine and provides me with a calm, serene outlook most of the time."

Yoga therapists and psychotherapists in the United States are reporting on the beneficial effects of treating both veterans and survivors of the World Trade Center attack suffering from the symptoms of PTSD. Psychotherapist Kirsten Trabbic Michels, a Yoga teacher and Phoenix Rising Yoga Therapist who used Yogic techniques—postures, breathing exercises, and guided visualizations—with Vietnam vets in a V.A. hospital in Maryland, says, "Although most of the men were initially reluctant to participate in something as foreign as Yoga, slowly many veterans came to appreciate the benefits they could receive. Veterans reported the breathing exercises provided an instantaneous experience of regaining control when they were feeling panicked or threatened. The body awareness gained through asana practice taught them how to relax muscle groups while simultaneously increasing strength and balance."[7] Most of the vets were in their fifties and had not taken care of themselves for thirty years. In addition to the many health problems they faced, many of them hated their bodies and were therefore wary of practicing postures with a psychotherapist and Yoga teacher in her twenties. The vets' initial resistance melted away as they began to see their Yoga sessions as "a forum for them to feel whatever it was that they were feeling—grief, anger, fear and pride and patriotism." The most powerful aspect of the work for Kirsten was in creating a container where as a group the veterans could feel safe enough to sit with whatever feelings were present for them.

Mercedes A. McCormick is a psychologist and Yoga therapist in private practice in the New York/New Jersey area. Dr. McCormick specializes in integrative psychotherapy and has been using Yogic practices—meditation, postures, and guided visualizations—with New Yorkers, both children and adults, suffering from the emotional impact of the terrorist attacks. Participants in the workshops she has conducted in New York City with adults affected by the events of September 11, 2001, express relief and gratitude for the practical tools they learn to handle stress. Often people suffering from PTSD are treated with antidepressants. "Introducing Yoga," says Dr. McCormick, "can be an effective way of reducing or perhaps even eliminating the need for medication and can help in the process of withdrawing from medication." Yoga and Yoga therapy "encourages the exploration of thoughts, feelings, body sensations, and behaviors related to traumatic events in a safe, supportive environment, recharging and healing the body and mind and helping to restore it to a condition of harmony and balance."[8]

If you are suffering from PTSD, don't wait to finish reading this book to find a Yoga class. Not only will the postures and breathing exercises help you, but the safe and soothing environment of the class will bring you solace. If, however, your disorder prevents you from feeling comfortable in a group setting, then contact a Yoga teacher for private sessions and invest in a video- or audiotape to practice at home.

Dysthymia

> The weather of Depression is unmodulated, its light a brownout.
>
> —WILLIAM STYRON, *Darkness Visible*[9]

For three years, Elizabeth knew that something beyond the pain she was feeling in her joints was wrong, but she didn't know what it was. A forty-one-year-old art historian, she remembered a time when she rode her bike nearly every day, when she had a circle of women friends with whom she went salsa dancing at a Latin club on Friday nights, when she went to sleep with a new idea for an exhibit at the museum where she was a curator and woke up already writing the catalogue copy in her head. But for the last three years, her bike had leaned against the wall with a flat tire and her friends had fallen away—some married, her best friend moved to Seattle, and the others, well, she didn't know about the others. Her phone didn't ring anymore. She stopped dancing when her physician diagnosed her aching joints as fibromyalgia and said she might have a degenerative arthritic condition in her spine.

When Elizabeth's mother died unexpectedly of a heart attack, she watched her younger sister go to pieces at the funeral and wondered why she didn't cry—why, in fact, she felt nothing. But though she didn't mourn her mother, she had trouble getting out of bed and was often late for work or called in sick. She decided to take a leave of absence from the museum to work on her medical problems and never went back. The money her mother had left her paid off the mortgage and covered most of her monthly expenses, and she added a little extra with occasional freelance writing assignments. Though she had enjoyed decorating her house when she'd bought it seven years earlier, it had now fallen into disrepair. She didn't call the plumber when her toilet leaked, and the hard wood of her bathroom floor darkened and warped. She rarely changed her sheets and almost never made the bed. Most of the time, her shutters stayed closed against the Arizona sun, and when her dishwasher and then her disposal broke down, she didn't bother to have them fixed.

Six months later, while walking her black Lab through the desert wash, she met an attractive man walking a golden retriever and they struck up a conversation. Sometimes she spoke with Tom when she saw him with his dog, and he seemed genuinely interested in her. When he asked her to dinner, she told him she was busy. But he persisted, and eventually they began to go out. He told her that he'd been married to a trial attorney, a woman he said was often angry, critical, and domineering. He said he appreciated Elizabeth's quiet demeanor, her soft voice, her willingness to go along with just about anything he wanted to do. But as they became better acquainted, he complained about her lack of energy, especially her lack of enthusiasm for sex. "There's no joy in your life," he told her one day when she said she was too tired to go to a basketball game with him. When he broke up with her, he said he'd been mistaken—that what he'd perceived as contentment and inner peace was, he thought, depression, and it was dragging him down.

Elizabeth didn't grieve much over the breakup, though she did cry a little when she saw him in the wash several weeks later, walking his dog with another woman. Mostly, she felt numb. As time passed, she let her dishes pile up in the sink and along the counter. Mail spilled off the kitchen table and onto her chairs. There were days when she left her dog in the fenced-in backyard and didn't leave the house. A trip to the grocery store seemed overwhelming.

Then her younger sister called to say she was coming for a visit, and Elizabeth made an effort. She called a cleaning service and a repairman for the broken-down appliances. She changed her sheets, made her bed, and had highlights put in her hair. She shopped for food she hadn't bothered to cook in years—salmon filets, artichokes, avocados, mangos, strawberries—and even arranged fresh flowers for the table. But the clean house and the new hairstyle couldn't hide the lack of energy, the slumped shoulders, her forced and artificial laughter at her sister's humor.

When her sister, as Tom had done, asked if she was depressed, Elizabeth denied it. "I don't feel sad," she said. "I never even cry."

"What do you feel?" her sister asked.

"Nothing."

"That's depression."

For the first time, Elizabeth admitted that, yes, maybe she was depressed.

When depression manifests in tears, we know that the emotional body is out of balance. But what about when there are no tears and we don't even feel the normal sadness when someone close to us dies? Sometimes, like Elizabeth, when we deny depression, it shows up in our bodies as physical symptoms—aches and pains that rise out of nowhere and often recede when we receive treatment for depression. Many of us may not recognize our depression until the people we love don't want to be around us anymore, or someone who loves us puts a name to what we feel.

In fact, Elizabeth was suffering from a kind of chronic depression called dysthymia. Like a low-grade fever that never goes away, dysthymia colors our perceptions about the world. A person suffering from dysthymia can function in her job, may have friends and relationships and what may appear to be a satisfying life. The sufferer may hardly be aware of the absence of joy in her life, because most likely, she's rarely known anything else. She may speak softly, her breath may be shallow, and her shoulders may slump. Her lack of zest and enthusiasm seem almost a natural outgrowth of her personality. To be clinically diagnosed as dysthymic, a person has to have three to five of the following symptoms for a period of at least two years:

Persistent sad, anxious, or empty mood

Loss of interest or pleasure in activities, including sex

Restlessness, irritability, or excessive crying

Feelings of guilt, worthlessness, helplessness, hopelessness, pessimism

Sleeping too much or too little

Appetite and/or weight loss or overeating and weight gain

Decreased energy, fatigue; feeling slowed down

Thoughts of death or suicide

Difficulty concentrating, remembering, or making decisions

Persistent physical symptoms that do not respond to treatment, such as headaches, digestive disorders, and chronic pain

The Gunas

In Yogic terms, Elizabeth was out of balance, suffering from a Tamasic depression. In Yogic science, three basic archetypes, known as the *gunas*, categorize our basic psychological states. If you are feeling in balance, neither depleted nor supercharged, you are in a *sattvic* (balanced) state. If you are out of balance, feeling lethargic and hopeless, then you are in a *tamasic* (inertia) state. Most people who are suffering from dysthymia or major depression are in a tamasic state. If, on the other hand, you are feeling too much energy, are nervous and anxious, you are in a *rajasic* (aggression) state. People who are suffering from anxiety-based depression or mania are in a rajasic state. All of the practices of Yoga are meant to bring your physical and emotional body into balance, or *sattva*. Some practices create more energy, leading you from a tamasic state back into balance. Others soothe and calm the excessive energy in your system, leading you from a rajasic state back into balance. This is why it's important to understand your depression, so that you can, with the help of a qualified teacher, design a practice that will be most balancing (sattvic) for you.

Source of Imbalance

Some people, like Elizabeth, have current situations that activate their depression. For others, there may be no apparent cause in their current life situation, yet they struggle with feelings of hopelessness and have little energy for their ordinary daily activities. What is the source of such a joyless life? For some, it may be a genetic predisposition. There are families in which alcoholism and depression have killed off family members for generations. For others, there may be a biochemical imbalance, perhaps inherited, perhaps due to deprivation, abuse, or neglect in early childhood. It is often difficult to distinguish a depression that is biochemically determined from one that is due to environmental factors, and different individuals respond to the same events differently. "Some children thrive despite early losses," says clinical psychologist George Goldman. "But if someone has a genetic predisposition toward depression," Goldman says, "even if the objective experience was a happy childhood, looking back, his subjective experience will be that he was unhappy."

On the other hand, there is strong evidence suggesting that our earliest experiences with our primary caregivers color our emotional experience throughout our lives. "Love, and the lack of it, change the young brain forever," say the authors of *A General Theory of Love.*[10] In fact, lack of human touch and sound is fatal to infants. One study showed that babies separated from their mothers and reared in orphanages during the 1940s, when it was thought unhygienic to handle them, lost weight, and despite being protected from infectious organisms, many of them died. Those who survived exhibited symptoms of depression. As noted in Chapter One, research with rhesus monkeys in the 1980s showed that when baby monkeys were separated from their mothers, they developed the symptoms of depression, and what's more, their biochemistry was altered.[11] "It is now assumed that depression may result from a complex interaction between genetic predisposition to the illness and early untoward life events such as child abuse or neglect," say the authors of a recent study on the neurobiology of depression. Such interactions induce significant changes in the central nervous system. The study goes on to suggest that changes to the brain's neuronal pathways persist into adulthood, "leading to a hypersensitive stress response system," which creates a "neurobiological vulnerability to depression and anxiety."[12]

Balancing the Imbalance

Whatever the source of the depressive feelings, Yoga can help. Elizabeth has found that a slow, gentle practice with longer holdings that also includes some dynamic movements and energizing breathing exercises works best to alleviate her symptoms. On the other hand, some people respond best to a more active practice. (In Chapter Five, we will look more closely at which kind of practice might be most effective for particular forms of depression.) As Elizabeth's teacher, I observe a significant difference in her appearance and her ability to connect with others when she's practicing and when she isn't. A tall, thin woman, when she walks into class after a period of absence, she is hunched forward with her head lowered, as though, if she could make herself small enough, no one would notice she's come back. She has trouble breathing deeply into the bottom of her lungs and often sits with her eyes closed while the rest of the class is taking deep belly breaths. But during the times she is able to come to class regularly, there is a visible change in her bearing. Her posture is better, she looks me straight in the eye, and I suddenly notice how attractive she is.

The mother hen in me would like to call her at six A.M. every morning to invite her to class. But all I can do is be present for her when she does show up. And her experience in class is always varied. "Sometimes I come out feeling peaceful," she says, "sometimes energized and alert, sometimes desperately sad. But I rarely come out feeling dead or anxious, my usual 'presentations' of depression. Yoga short-circuits the downward spiral for me—makes me feel less hateful toward my body, mind, and emotions." While I believe that a regular daily practice would make a difference in the way Elizabeth manages her dysthymia, I trust her when she tells me that her mat is "my little island of calm presence, even if I just sit on it."

Bipolar Disorder

> And then my blue funk passed. Passed? It shot by me like a rocket
> and dragged me with it. I started sailing.
>
> —JOSHUA LOGAN, *Josh*[13]

While Elizabeth suffered from a general lack of energy and feeling, others may experience a type of depression called bipolar disorder, or manic depression, characterized by periods of depression alternating with episodes of excessive energy and activity. In Yogic terms, the person in a manic episode would be experiencing a rajasic state. He may feel so euphoric that he doesn't believe he is ill. His mood is abnormally elevated, he needs little sleep, and his racing thoughts and rapid speech make him feel brilliant to himself and sometimes even to others. A milder form of this disorder is cyclothymia, a condition in which a person may have elevated energy and some of the same symptoms of mania for an extended period of time, during which she may be unusually productive, followed by feelings of depression. According to Kay Redfield Jamison, a psychiatrist and author of a book about manic depression, *Touched with Fire,* one person in three who has cyclothymia will develop "full syndrome depression, hypomania or mania."[14] Jamison, who suffers from bipolar disorder herself, points out that most people who have manic-depressive illness "maintain their reason and their ability to function personally and professionally" most of the time.

Many of our finest poets, artists, writers, composers, and creative thinkers have suffered from manic-depressive illness. The list is long and familiar—Anne Sexton, Sylvia Plath, Charles Baudelaire, John Berryman, Samuel Taylor Coleridge, William Faulkner, Mary Shelley, Louise Bogan, Walt Whitman, Ernest Hemingway, F. Scott Fitzgerald, Virginia Woolf, Tennessee Williams, William Blake, and Ezra Pound, to name just a few of the writers. Someone in a manic episode has a marked increase in energy and activity but can also become irritable and impatient. Their delusions of grandeur often cause them to be intolerant of lesser mortals who might attempt to interrupt their flights of brilliant speech. Leonard Woolf describes such an episode when Virginia Woolf was in the manic phase of her illness: "She talked almost without stopping for two or three days, paying no attention to anyone in the room or anything said to her. For almost a day what she said was coherent; the sentences meant something, though it was nearly all wildly insane. Then gradually it became completely incoherent, a mere jumble of dissociated words."[15]

But the finer aspects of mania—the increased energy, the rapid speech, the flight of ideas—may fit a fertile and creative period in an artist's life. In the novel *Solstice,* Joyce Carol Oates describes the onset of a manic burst of creativity in the life of the abstract painter Sheila Trask. If you read this as though you are inside a manic episode, you will see that Oates's style mirrors the chaos in the character's mind:

> Sheila was in one of her ecstatic high-flying moods; Sheila was in one of her dull-eyed stupefied moods, exhausted, grainy-skinned, not very attractive. She spent her mornings driving about the country roads, she spent her mornings on the telephone, suddenly there was a houseguest at Edgemont (a relative? a cousin?), suddenly she turned up at Monica's, carrying a bag of groceries, goat's-milk cheese and Norwegian rye crackers, that very same country pâté she loved to gorge on, and two six-packs of imported German beer. God she was hungry!—famished!
>
> Another thing, too: the way the days passed, spun, a sun and a moon and a sun again, zip and it's through: you get the point where you sit hypnotized by the clock, any fucking clock, watching the hands move, forgetting to breathe.
>
> Did Monica understand?
>
> And there were the mirror-ghouls, the mirror-leeches.
>
> "Sisters" of a sort. Whom you don't recognize though they seem to recognize you.
>
> *Did* Monica understand?[16]

Often mania is accompanied by a state of hypersexuality. At a spiritual retreat a few years ago, I met an intelligent man who had been a spiritual seeker for many years, practicing various forms of meditation and, he later told me, his own version of Tantric sex. People who suffer from manic depression live for months without experiencing mood swings. This was the case when I met Jeff, and I did not realize he suffered from manic depression until he told me he did. He described episodes in his life when he had believed he was invincible and had tried to fly from window ledges and scale buildings, times he had committed crimes and been arrested. We talked often during the retreat, and I thought him an intelligent and sensitive man, aware of his disorder and managing it well. However, several months later, I received a long, rambling letter from him, inviting me to join a group of very young women whom he believed he was helping toward enlightenment with his blessed semen. I assumed from the letter that Jeff had stopped taking his medication.

The person in the midst of a manic episode often feels so powerful, so energized, that she is not likely to seek treatment, while those around her may be confused and unsure. In Oates's novel, Sheila Trask finishes the paintings for a major one-woman show in what seems to be the midst of a manic episode. But eventually, in most cases of mania, family members or friends are forced to seek help when poor judgment leads to inappropriate social behavior and activities that put the person suffering from mania and the lives of others at risk.

In 1990, after her second hospitalization for bipolar disorder, forty-one-year-old Penny Smith was told that she could expect to be in and out of psychiatric hospitals for the rest of her life. Her family had a history of bipolar disorder on both sides. Her paternal grandmother committed suicide. Her maternal grandfather, who suffered rages and was alcoholic, was most likely bipolar. Her maternal grandmother and one of her sisters are bipolar, and her daughter Peggy, now fourteen, was diagnosed with the disorder when she was eight. "Manic depressive illness is a genetic disease," says Kay Redfield Jamison, "running strongly, not to say pervasively, in some families while absent in most,"[17] and Penny's family clearly illustrates the strong genetic link. The role of genes in affective disorders is underscored by the fact that if one identical twin has manic-depressive illness, the other is likely (70 to 100 percent) to have it as well.

Before her last hospitalization, Penny was frequently awake throughout the night, painting and stenciling the walls of her house, pulling weeds outside by flashlight, and hallucinating images of spiders and bugs. As a rapid cycler, Penny swung from intense mania to the depths of depression many times during the day. She tried eleven medications, including lithium, but nothing worked and she entered a treatment center. Soon after her release, Penny learned a few Kripalu-style Yoga postures and breathing exercises from her daughter's preschool teacher. As her practice increased from three days a week to nearly every day, the intensity and length of her episodes of mania and depression diminished, and she was gradually able to develop an awareness that in Yoga is referred to as "Witness Consciousness." Her mood swings didn't disappear immediately, but she began to sense when she was headed into depression or mania and was able to take better care of herself. Eventually, with regular practice and one medication, Celexa, her lifelong pattern of severe mood swings ended. In the twelve years that Penny has been practicing Hatha Yoga, she has not been hospitalized again.

The first symptom to disappear as a result of the pranayama breathing techniques Penny learned was the panic attacks. Those breathing techniques are simple enough that Penny was able to teach them to her then eight-year-old daughter, so that she, too, could begin to manage her attacks. "No one can possibly have panic attacks while concentrating on her breath," Penny says. "Through Yoga, I realized that I had been doing shallow breathing most of my life."

The breath was not the only aspect of her practice that made a significant difference early on in managing her illness. Practicing the postures helped her become more aware of her body, so that when she felt tension developing in a particular area, she was able to release it with a specific posture. Penny's practice begins with a series of stretches that warm the body slowly, and she follows this with an energizing sequence of standing poses, which she holds for at least thirty seconds. Next she practices backbends, then ends her practice with two gentle restorative postures, one of which is a supported backbend described in the Yoga Experience at the end of this chapter. The other is an inversion. An inversion is an upside-down posture in which the blood flow in your body is reversed. Penny's inverted posture is a supported Shoulderstand. You will learn more about the physiological and psychological benefits of inverted postures in the next chapter. The restorative poses balance the more active portion of her practice, so that when she's finished she feels both energized and calm.

And meditation has helped her too. "When I was depressed, one negative thought would lead to the next in a vicious cycle. Through meditation techniques, I'm able to let go of the ongoing negative thoughts that come with depression." When her thoughts are racing, she uses mantra meditation. She feels it's important to use the same mantra each time she meditates. "My mind has become so attuned to the mantra 'so hum' that it quickly takes me to a deep level." When she wakes up in the middle of the night, Penny uses this mantra along with calming pranayama breathing exercises to fall back to sleep.

Recently Penny's equanimity has been seriously challenged by divorce. After twenty-six years of marriage, her husband left and moved across the country. During the hardest times at the end of their relationship, she says it was her practice that kept her sane. Despite this major loss in her life and the fact that she must face the complexities of raising a bipolar daughter alone, Penny Smith finds balance every day on her Yoga mat. "I am alive today because of Kripalu Yoga," she says, "which focuses on the internal aspect of the practice. Every sensation is sacred and responded to with tenderness. Kripalu means compassion, and that's what I needed."

Given the genetic predisposition in Penny's family and her probable biochemistry, she and her daughter are likely "hardwired" for bipolar disorder. Penny has learned how to manage her symptoms, reducing her mood swings and panic attacks, so that her life works. But she will never be entirely free of the disorder. If you are genetically programmed to be depressed, Yoga cannot change your DNA. However, in such cases, Yoga can help you control your symptoms and manage your life.

Not everyone is hardwired in the same way as Penny, or has the same experience of bipolar depression. Julia, a thirty-four-year-old former ballerina, writer, and mother diagnosed as bipolar, does not have a family history of the disorder. In her case, symptoms emerged six years ago, after the birth of her first child. Julia began practicing Yoga only after her last manic episode ten months ago, and is just beginning to feel the effects of her regular (though not daily) practice on her mood swings. "If I don't practice Yoga for a few days, I find myself retreating to those edgy feelings that cause my mood to swing wildly up or down. My husband jokes that he 'sends' me to Yoga class to get 'rebalanced.'" Exactly! Her husband may not be familiar with the principle of the gunas, and how her practice naturally brings Julia into a more sattvic state, but he is the happy recipient of her more balanced mood.

Like those of many people suffering from manic depression, Julia's episodes of mania and depression are cyclical and seasonal. She has her worst times during the latter part of her menstrual cycle and overall in the spring/summer. Since her last manic episode was just last spring, she has not yet gone through a vulnerable period while practicing Yoga. However, she has noticed that her periods of depression have lightened. "It almost seems as if I can 'leech' the depression out of me as I concentrate on my breathing in the various postures."

Julia began studying ballet when she was five years old, so she has been aware of her body for most of her life. But as a satisfying form of self-expression, dancing had become impossible for her, because it brought back memories of failure and competition. "It's great for me that I've found another mode of expression that is just as concerned about alignment and balance but that focuses not on how graceful you look in the mirror, but on the inner grace that can grow from a heartfelt practice."

Major Depressive Episode

> I did not hear the bird sounds.
> They had left.
> I did not see the speechless clouds,
> I saw only the little white dish of my faith
> Breaking in the crater.
>
> —ANNE SEXTON, "The Sickness Unto Death,"
> *That Awful Rowing Toward God*[18]

If we practice enough sun salutations, if we sit in Lotus Pose gazing at a candle flame for twenty minutes every day, if we volunteer at a soup kitchen, if we try all the practices this book recommends, will we feel better? Well, maybe. Even probably. But if it's one A.M. in your own personal dark night of the soul, if you're in a major depressive episode and the thought of getting dressed in the morning is more than you can bear, you aren't likely to have the energy or the courage to get out of bed, let alone let your heart lead you in a forward bend with arms widespread.

If you are in the midst of a major depressive episode, you may suffer from the same list of symptoms as someone whose mood is dysthymic, but in a much more severe form, so that your normal functioning is impaired. People suffering from major depression have difficulty main-taining relationships, doing their work, even accomplishing everyday tasks, and the shame they feel compounds the effect of the depression. In his eloquent account of his own experience with depression, *Darkness Visible,* William Styron writes that his state of mind was virtually "inde-scribable" and that someone who has never experienced this anguish cannot possibly comprehend the actual dimensions of this suffering. "Such incomprehension," he says, "has usually been due not to a failure of sympathy but to the basic inability of healthy people to imagine a form of torment so alien to everyday experience."[19]

If you are in a severe depression, you may need an allopathic approach—medication, even time in a hospital or treatment center—before you can even begin to think about sitting with your spine erect, your sitting bones grounded, your crown lifted, breathing Yogic Three-Part Breath. On the other hand, if you're in a place that admits no light, there *are* Yoga practices that may crack through the fog of even a major depressive episode. I'll describe in Chapter Seven a specific breathing technique that has demonstrated as high as a 73 percent recovery rate from major depressive episodes, a rate that nearly equals that achieved with electroconvulsive therapy (ECT).

But whether you follow a psychopharmacological approach or choose an alternative treatment (as do millions of Americans), you're going to get onto your Yoga mat quicker if you accept where you are. What if you could make peace with your depressed mood? When you can embrace the darkness, you're one step closer to the light. "What if 'depression' were simply a state of being," asks Thomas Moore in *Care of the Soul*, "neither good nor bad, something the soul does in its own good time and for its own good reasons?"[20] "The best protection against this pain," says Bernadette Roberts in *The Experience of No-Self*, "is to fully accept it; by virtually sinking into it, sinking into the feeling of utter misery and nothingness, the pain loses much of its punch."[21] But what does accepting depression look like? Does it mean you stay in bed all day, avoiding others, in your effort not to resist the depression? Perhaps a mental health day is precisely what is called for. But true acceptance is itself a practice to be cultivated as you would any other specific tech-nique. Even as you're hibernating from the world, if you can plan one small practice, you might let just enough light in that staying in bed feels uncomfortable. And that one small practice, done regularly, may balance the brain chemistry in ways that make the depression tolerable.

We may not cure the major depression episode with our practice, but we may begin to accept these times in our lives and be able to grow from what Moore says are "the gifts of soul that only depression can provide."[22] I know—when you're in it, it hardly feels like a gift. Feelings of hopelessness seem to offer little nourishment to the soul. But if you can accept your suffering, even for a few moments, you may begin to build a container of peace in which the depression can be observed. "I really wasn't good for anything anymore except surrender," writes novelist Tom Farrington in a moving account of his own depression. "For perhaps five minutes a day, my fevered brain would cool into acceptance, and I would grow calm and peaceful, reconciled to my nothingness.

"The embrace of a fathomless nothingness is not exactly the American Dream," Farrington goes on to say. "There's still not a damn thing you can see worth doing in the whole wide world. It's just that you've made your peace with this."[23]

Learning Love and Acceptance

Several years ago, I lost someone dear to me—Louise, a woman who, since I was three, had been like a second mother to me. More than anyone else, she believed in me as a writer. The day I learned that she died, I also received a rejection letter from an editor whose press had been seriously considering my novel-in-progress for publication. For weeks, grief, failure, and self-doubt were the vessels through which all my experiences poured. My sleep was disrupted, my Yoga practice became compulsive and driven, and I found it difficult to meditate. I experienced dark shifts in mood, a lack of energy, and an inability to focus even during my own practice. But while I was teaching Yoga, I felt centered, calm, and at home in my body. As I encouraged my students to cultivate love and acceptance for their bodies, without judgment about their limitations, I returned to the sense of contentment (*samtosha*) that my practice had opened to me over the years. The language I used to guide my students in class was language I needed to hear, especially at this time of grief and perceived failure in my life. It was the language of acceptance.

My beloved child, break your heart no longer. Each time you judge yourself, you break your own heart. When I first heard these words, attributed to Swami Kripalvanandji, in a Yoga class at Kripalu in 1989, I felt something soften and relax inside. I realized that the tight knots of self-criticism I'd tied myself into had formed roadblocks on the interior path to liberation. Over the years, as I heard myself repeating those words to my students in Yoga classes, those knots began to dissolve and I was able to reduce, though not entirely eliminate, the level of anxiety about who I was and how I showed up in the world. Mostly, since I began a daily Yoga practice, I've felt abundant and whole, better than at any other time in my life. But when my novel was rejected, that tiny petri dish of self-doubt inside was fertilized. Maybe I didn't deserve to succeed. If only I'd worked harder, revised the novel another time, changed the title, stayed married, done more therapy, memorized Patanjali's *Yoga Sutras,* dealt more consciously with my relationship problems . . . STOP!!! *My beloved child, break your heart no longer. Each time you judge yourself, you break your own heart.*

When I sat, legs crossed in half-lotus with my Yoga students, all the self-battering chatter stopped. I listened to the words I used. I heard myself inviting my students to let go of their expectations about how they were supposed to show up, on and off the mat, to release any clinging thoughts about the past or the future, to let go of the obstacles that kept them from experiencing the free flow of thoughts and feelings in the present moment. I invited my students to rest in the flow of breath coming in and out through the tips of their nostrils, and I rested with them. During the weeks after Louise's death and my novel was returned to me, my experience as a Yoga teacher, truly teaching what I needed to learn about self-acceptance, saying out loud the words I needed to hear in order to love myself, was the greatest gift I could give myself.

No matter what form of depression you may suffer from, love and acceptance are the two essential elements necessary in developing control over your symptoms. Cultivating both will, over time, allow you to manage your symptoms and have a happier life. Eventually, you may feel completely recovered. Both self-love and self-acceptance grow with practice. All of the practitioners I interviewed for this chapter owe their improvement, in part, to their growing ability, through the practice of Yoga, to accept themselves no matter how chaotic or tormented their mental state. "Self-love," says Richard Miller, "is not a resignation or a blind acceptance of your symptoms. It's a freedom from self-loathing."

But how, after a lifetime spent listening to your inner critic, of judging yourself too harshly, of feeling ashamed because you suffer from depression, do you suddenly begin to love yourself? Self-acceptance isn't automatic just because your Yoga teacher encourages you to love yourself. It doesn't happen just because you repeat affirmations. Learning to love yourself happens slowly, over time. Affirmations and gentle reminders from someone who isn't afraid of your symptoms—a therapist, a Yoga teacher, a beloved, a good friend—can help. The first step may be finding the right Yoga class, where the teacher is less concerned about the exact accomplishment of the posture and more concerned with the healthy relationship you are developing with your body.

Cultivating Self-Awareness

In *The Yoga Sutras*, Patanjali says, "By study of scriptures and of oneself, the consciousness is united with the desired or loved divinity."[24] Or as modern Yogis have put it, "The highest spiritual practice is self-awareness without judgment." Before you can clear the way to communion with the divine, you must acknowledge and move beyond the obstacles to the free flow of thought and feeling. Depression is an obstacle to that free flow. If you are willing to take a step back and observe your mood, you are practicing self-awareness. From here, you can better manage and even overcome your depression by developing a practice that suits your feelings. Whether you feel anxious and active in your depression (*rajasic*) or fogged in and passive (*tamasic*), understanding the subtleties of your state of mind is important.

Are there manic aspects to your depression? Is your depression accompanied by anxiety? Or are you feeling listless and depleted? This understanding is vital if you are going to meet the depression where you are. An active, anxious mind will reject any attempt to immediately relax. And a mind numbed by melancholia will reject any attempt to suddenly perk up. "Meeting the depression," says Miller, "means hanging out in the chaos and then slowly introducing alternatives." He compares this strategy to handling a young child who's grabbed a sharp knife off the kitchen counter. You don't want to grab it back and risk injury to him or to yourself. Instead, you distract him from the danger of the knife with something equally shiny, perhaps, but safer. So, in Yoga, we "offer the mind a bone," says Miller. This may take the form of a sound, perhaps a Sanskrit mantra or tone, or perhaps a saying.

Affirmations for Overcoming Depression

Here's a bone I like to offer my mind first thing in the morning, before I rise from my bed. I find that it soothes my heart and cultivates a feeling of gratitude. And gratitude, in my experience, lightens the heart and eases me into my day. As you inhale, say to yourself, "Thou art with me." As you exhale, repeat to yourself, "Thank you." Do this as often as you wish for as long as you wish, but at least three times in a row. If using a formal "Thou art" is not comfortable, try substituting "You are." If the notion of divinity troubles you, feel free to change the first phrase to "I am not alone." A good place to practice is in bed, before you go to sleep, then again in the morning before you rise.

Affirmation for Self-Acceptance

Here is a simple set of affirmations that may help when you are feeling low. You may practice this while sitting on a meditation cushion or in a chair, or at your desk in the middle of a hectic day. Close your eyes. As you inhale through your nostrils, say to yourself, "I am not my depressed mood." Hold your breath for four counts. Exhale slowly and repeat to yourself, "I am," six times. Repeat this sequence at least three times. You may change the first phrase to reflect what you are feeling in the moment—for example: "I am not this anxious mood," or "I am not these confused thoughts," or "I am not the chaos I am feeling." Always end with the repetition of "I am."

yoga experience

I've included two postures or posture sequences here. The first practice will activate, the second will calm and soothe. You can determine which order to do them in, based on what you have ascertained about your state of mind during the meditation at the end of the last chapter. If you are feeling sluggish and weak, start with the soothing practice and move to the activating practice. If you are feeling too much energy, begin with the activating practice and move to the soothing practice.

Activating: Flying Cow

This is a four-part sequence, adapted from a Viniyoga sequence suggested by Gary Kraftsow in *Yoga for Wellness: Healing with the Timeless Teachings of Viniyoga*.[25] John DeCoville was practicing this sequence when he had the breakthrough that enabled him to accept his grief.

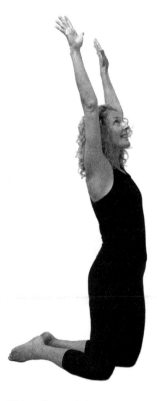

1. Come into a high kneeling position, knees hip-width apart. As you inhale, raise your arms over your head. Feel yourself lifted up internally. Imagine that you can lift the bottom of your heart. Smile into your heart. Put a soft smile on your face. Let your eyes roll up behind their lids.

2. As you exhale, come forward onto your forearms with your tailbone lifted.

Flying Cow: Inhale your arms up

3. As you inhale, rise onto your palms in a table position, with your tailbone lifted and your crown lifted. Your pelvis is tilted up and back; your belly hammocks down and out of the pelvis; your heart is lifted, your shoulders are drawn back; your eyes are rolled up behind their lids. Hold the breath.

4. As you exhale, round the spine like a cat, draw the belly back to the spine, the chin to the chest, and sink your hips on your heels, forehead on the mat, with your arms extended.

Repeat the sequence no more than eight times.

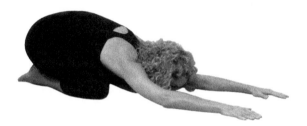

Flying Cow: Exhale onto forearms

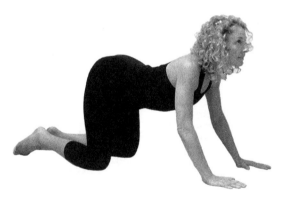

Flying Cow: Inhale to table position

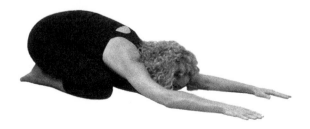

Flying Cow: Exhale hips to heels

5.   As you inhale, "fly up," returning to your original high kneeling position with your arms over your head.

Repeat this sequence up to eight times. When you have finished, sit for a moment on your heels, your hands folded in your lap, and observe what you're feeling in your physical body and your emotional body. You may feel a lightness in your solar plexus and an expanded, open feeling in your heart. Let the energy circulate throughout your body.

Calming: Smiling Heart Pose

This is a supported backbend that feels wonderful after a stressful day. It's one of Penny Smith's favorite poses to do at the end of her practice, and it's highly recommended for depression by many Yoga traditions. I call this "Smiling Heart Pose." It requires several props.

1.   Place two folded blankets, a bolster, or a firm cushion under your back, just beneath your shoulder blades. Make sure the lift is comfortable and modify if you need to, using more or less support as feels right for your body.

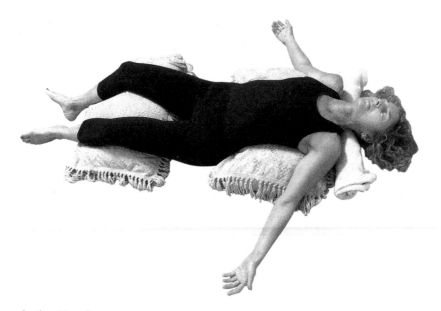

Smiling Heart Pose

2. Place a rolled blanket or towel underneath your neck so that the back of your head rests comfortably on the mat.

3. Place a bolster or cushion under your knees and allow your legs to be a comfortable (usually about hip-width) distance apart.

4. Allow your arms to stretch comfortably out at shoulder level, with your palms facing up.

You may also wish to use an eyebag in this position. Stay in this position for at least five minutes, practicing the breath described below. To make this posture more stimulating, try lifting your arms over your head on the floor behind you.

Breath: Yogic Three-Part Breath (Dirga Pranayama)

Yogic Three-Part Breath can be done in a seated posture but is most easily learned in a lying-down position. It is a good breath to practice while in the Smiling Heart Pose, discussed above. It is also an excellent breath with which to relax before sleep. This pranayama gets breath moving fully through the lungs. It's a good way to release tensions stored in the body. You may wish to use your hands in the beginning so you can feel the breath moving into and expanding the three separate areas of your lungs. Place both hands on your abdomen, above and below your navel. Relax your belly. As you inhale through the nostrils, feel your lower lungs filling like a balloon, and notice how your belly rises into your hands. Practice breathing fully and deeply into your lower lungs for several breaths. Next, keep one hand on your belly and place the other at the bottom of your rib cage. After filling your lower lungs and inflating your belly, fill your middle lungs so that your rib cage expands and you feel your hand rising on your chest. Practice breathing in this way for several breaths. Next, keep one hand on your belly and move the other hand to the base of your throat. Inhale fully, filling the lower lungs and the middle lungs, then bring the breath into the upper lungs and feel your upper chest expanding into your hand. As you exhale, first deflate your upper lungs, your middle lungs, then your lower lungs, as though you're pouring the breath out like a glass of water. Once you are comfortable with the breath, bring your arms to the sides of your body with the palms faceup or, if you are sitting, with your palms faceup on your knees.

To make this breathing exercise slightly more stimulating, try holding your breath at the top of the inhalation for no more than four counts. Release the breath for six counts. The slow release is calming, and you will stay in balance.

You can stay in this position, breathing Yogic Three-Part Breath, for at least five minutes but not more than fifteen. If you are in Smiling Heart Pose, come out slowly, using your hands for support, as you roll to your right side and sit up. Sit for a few moments, noticing how you feel in your physical body and your emotional body.

why yoga works

I know a cure for sadness:
Let your hands touch something that
makes your eyes
smile.

—MIRABAI[1]

Life-Changing Practice

Yoga is so much a part of my daily life now, creating an everyday sense of well-being, that it is only when I *don't* practice that I notice the effects. A kind of lethargy settles into my limbs early in the day. If I haven't practiced Yoga in the morning, I may neglect to do other beneficial things as well, like ride my bike or call a friend. I may not feel as productive at my writing. I'm not surprised when a few standing postures and a couple of rounds of a rapid breathing exercise like Skull-Shining Breath (*Kapalabhati*) give me an energy boost. But, while I feel the loss of a welcome habit when I don't practice for just one day, people new to Yoga are often amazed at how good they feel when they do practice for just one day. "Life-changing," said Susan after her very first class.

On and off throughout her life, Susan has had many of the symptoms of dysthymia. Now a Phoenix postal carrier in her fifties, she was raised on a farm in Kansas, believing that "women were *who* they married." Because she didn't date much in high school, she often felt she would never measure up to her family's and community's expectations. Today she takes care of her aging mother, who doesn't believe in showing or talking about emotions. "I feel trapped, and though I try to look for the good that is coming from living with my mother, I find myself depressed about the situation." When she's depressed, Susan watches a lot of TV and cannot put her personal belongings away, living amid the clutter. "Most of my life I have struggled with being worthy of a wonderful, loving relationship." But a lasting love has eluded Susan. "When nobody called to ask me out, I felt like a failure." For many years, she masked her unhappiness with alcohol.

Three months ago, Susan began a regular practice of Yoga. She finds that the Yogic breathing exercises, especially Skull-Shining Breath (*Kapalabhati*), which is a *kriya* (complete action) that cleanses the system, and Alternate-Nostril Purifying Breath (*Nadi Sodhana*), which is a pranayama, can lift her mood. (You'll find a complete explanation of these breathing exercises and many more in Chapter Six.) In my private work with Susan, we designed a daily practice for her that incorporates a number of energizing breaths and postures done dynamically, using breath and repetition, to stimulate her energy. Susan was recently diagnosed with adult-onset diabetes II, so much of her personal practice is designed to stimulate and nourish the midsection of her body, in particular her pancreas, which is responsible for producing glucagons and insulin. Many of these poses are also good for her depression. "I feel like a new person after Yoga," she says. Since she began practicing, her depressed moods are not as intense. "I don't stay in the low place very long, and I have more energy. I am so grateful to have found this thing called Yoga. I truly believe it is a lifesaver for me. I am feeling so much better about myself already, and I know it is only going to get better."

The Eight-Limbed Path

When Susan began her Yoga practice, she was immediately reaping the benefits of at least five, possibly six, of the eight Yogic branches of the Yoga tree we talked about in Chapter One. I'm referring here to the Eight-Limbed Path, set down by Patanjali in *The Yoga Sutras*. When Patanjali compiled *The Yoga Sutras* in 200 C.E., the first written guidelines for the practice of Yoga postures, pranayamas, and meditation techniques, these principles had been transmitted orally from master to disciple for thousands of years. While what Patanjali recorded were guidelines for practice and not the practices themselves, which required a personal relationship between teacher and student, Patanjali set forth a kind of treatment plan to address the categories of mental and emotional distress. That plan is known as the Eight-Limbed Path (*ashta-anga*).

In *The Yoga Sutras,* Patanjali describes nine distractions, or obstacles, to inner awareness—disease, dullness, doubt, carelessness, laziness, addiction, false perception, failure to reach firm ground, and instability. He goes on to describe four pathological states that accompany these obstacles— depression, anxiety, trembling in the limbs, and unsteady breath. These states, he suggests, can be managed and even ameliorated with the following eight-part prescription: *yama* (restraint), *niyama* (observances), *asana,* (postures), *pranayama* (breath control), *pratyahara* (withdrawal of the senses), *dharana* (concentration), *dhyana* (absorption), and *samadhi* (cosmic consciousness). Susan knows little of Patanjali's prescription, but in her practice, she experiences the beneficial effects of stretching her body and compressing the glands in various postures (*asana*). She feels the immediate, energizing effects of rapid abdominal breathing, and the calming effects of slow, deep diaphragmatic breaths (*pranayama*). When she focuses her attention on the breath in our centering meditation, she is withdrawing her mind from the senses (*pratyahara*). When I guide her to use a mantra during the holding of a posture, she is concentrating (*dharana*). During that holding, if she follows the direction to stay in touch with the sensations in her body, her mind is absorbed (*dhyana*), and there may be times when, through the holding, or in the release of the posture, she has glimpses of a deeply healing state (*samadhi*). But Susan doesn't know any of these Sanskrit words, nor does she know she's involved in a systematic treatment for her depression. All Susan knows is that she feels good when she practices Yoga, and that's maybe all you need to know, too.

Short-Term Effects of Yoga

What is happening in Susan's body that is producing this feel-good response? A small Scandinavian study that measured brain waves before and after a two-hour Yoga class found that alpha waves (relaxation) and theta waves (unconscious memory, dreams, and emotions) increased by 40 percent.[2] The increase in alpha waves and theta waves measured in the Scandinavian study means that the brain is more deeply relaxed after Yoga and that the subjects have better contact with their subconscious and their emotions. Previous research has shown that depressed, introverted people typically have more alpha waves in the left frontal-temporal region, while optimistic, extroverted people have more alpha waves on the right. In the Scandinavian study, after the Yoga session, alpha waves increased in the right temporal lobe. That theta waves also increased supports the notion that Yoga works to alleviate depression not only by increasing brain chemicals that contribute to a feel-good response—endorphins, enkephalins, and serotonin—but also through greater access to feelings.

Susan may also feel good after Yoga because the stress hormone cortisol is reduced. Researchers at the Jefferson Medical College in Philadelphia, in cooperation with the Yoga Research Society, found that practitioners experienced a significant drop in cortisol levels after a single Yoga class.[3] In one study in France, when daily Yoga sessions were offered to hospitalized psychiatric patients, the authors of the study observed that "following the Yoga session, patients feel a sense of relaxation and mild euphoria, lasting for several hours. After eight to ten days of daily practice, certain physical symptoms may start to disappear. And after a period of one to two months, psychiatric symptoms may start to diminish."[4]

There is a large body of scientific evidence that demonstrates that physical exercise is effective in treating depression. A recent analytical review of the literature published in the *British Journal of Medicine* found that exercise treatments reduced depressive symptoms and are similar to psychotherapeutic or cognitive treatments in their effectiveness.[5]

Exercise alone creates beneficial physiological and psychological changes; however, study after study in India has shown that regular practice of Yoga accounts for more beneficial changes than does exercise. In one experiment, when three months of Yoga training were given to a group of forty physical education teachers who already had an average of 8.9 years physical training, significant improvements in general health were produced in terms of body weight and blood pressure reduction and improved lung functioning. "There was also evidence of decreased autonomic arousal, increased psychophysiological relaxation (heart rate and respiratory rate reduction), and improved somatic steadiness (decreased errors in the steadiness test)."[6] What this means is that the mind is focused and alert, ready to respond as in fight or flight, yet the body is relaxed and calm.

According to Dharma Singh Khalsa, M.D., a board-certified anesthesiologist specializing in anti-aging medicine and coauthor of the book *Meditation as Medicine,* Yoga and meditation can alter the very biochemistry of the brain more directly and efficiently than regular exercise. When you do Yoga stretching, you send a message through the spinal cord back to your brain that causes your brain chemistry to change. That "feel-good" sensation after Yoga practice arises from the balance of stimulation and relaxation you are providing your brain. "First of all, you are stimulating your pituitary gland to release endorphins. Your peripheral glandular system is producing adrenaline and norepenephrin-type compounds that travel to the brain and give you that mild stimulating effect. On the other hand, you are also stimulating a relaxation response." You feel more relaxed because your cortisol level drops, and you are increasing oxygen consumption and reducing muscle stiffness and tension. This is the balancing effect of the physical practice—the true union of energy and relaxation. That is why Susan feels so much better, even after just one session.

But you don't take an antidepressant medication just once and expect to feel better. You take it regularly. So with Yoga, to restore the body and mind to a steady state of well-being, you must also practice regularly. The very *commitment* to practice can begin to diminish depressive symptoms. Unlike taking a pill two or three times a day, when a Yoga student practices once a day, she is adding the element of what psychologists call "self-control"—the ability to be actively involved in the healing process. Self-control, not to be confused with willpower or restraint, means, in this context, that you can determine your own course of action. Self-control, as in self-determination, has been shown in numerous studies to have a positive outcome in recovery from illnesses, including depression.[7] Of all the ways that her regular practice has helped Susan, the element of self-control is one of the most crucial. "Yoga offers me the opportunity to practice something that I can do for myself and moves me from the paralyzing effects of depression."

Yoga Rx

Psychiatrist Roy King began his own Yoga practice in the late sixties while an undergraduate at Cornell. He has practiced on and off during the years he studied art history, earned a Ph.D. in mathematics, and attended medical school. When he became medical director of the Stanford Partial Hospitalization Program, it was a chance for him to explore his vision of using Yoga in the treatment plan for people suffering from mental illness. In the day program he directed, which treated people who had been hospitalized, mostly for depression, his curriculum included occupational therapy, group psychotherapy, art therapy, poetry therapy, and a Yoga class. He and his colleague led postures, a pranayama in which the breath was retained then slowly exhaled, and a concentration form of meditation. "People suffering from depression," says King, "lack motivation and often have an impaired ability to focus. So we tried to keep everything simple and clear. A lot of depressed people are stiff, so just getting them moving in a Yoga class helps to clarify their minds, so that they can more easily do the concentration exercise." The meditation was also simple. King would bring in an object like an orange or a seashell, and the group practiced an open-eyed concentration.

Everything was done to keep the class grounded, feeling the sensations in their bodies. Both King and an occupational therapist made every effort to keep the patients in touch with reality. King and his colleagues studied the effect of the various therapy groups. Self-reported stress levels, on a scale of one to ten, were measured before and after each group activity. As compared to poetry therapy and directed art therapy, Yoga practice significantly reduced the patients' feelings of stress.

Gland Stimulation

The traditional understanding of the *chakra* system is that there are seven (some traditions vary on this) vortices—or spinning wheels of energy—in the body, often graphically depicted as lotuses. I've always been amazed how the energy centers (chakras) in the body align so clearly with what we know about the major glands. Thousands of years before medical science isolated the major glands in the body and understood their function, Yogis were using postures, sounds, and visualizations to stimulate the chakras. Now we know that they were increasing the secretion of hormones responsible for our general well-being. "The glands are the guardians of health," says Dr. Khalsa. The hormones your glands produce in part determine your moods and your mode of thinking. On the other hand, your frame of mind affects your neurological system, which in turn affects your glandular system and endocrine system, which then affects the immune system. These systems, including your individual way of seeing the world, are totally interwoven. "By changing the secretions of the glands into the blood," says Khalsa, "you are creating a bloodstream with the right chemical milieu to nourish the brain, the rest of the body, and of course the immune system. Yoga in general, and Kundalini Yoga specifically, targets the glandular system with specific sounds and sequences of postures that compress the glands. The mantra sounds actually get the master glands of the brain— the pineal, the hypothalamus, and the pituitary glands—to secrete in a way that gives you a light, natural stimulation of the mind and body— the opposite of depression."

The Healing Role of Sound

In the Yoga of sound (*Nada Yoga*), there are a number of tones that are thought to specifically activate the various energy centers, to stimulate the brain and "resonate and harmonize with the innate vibrations of the universe."[8] Certainly research bears this out. In a recent study in Italy, scientists discovered that mantra and rosary repetition benefit the heart, and both prayer and mantra slow the breath rate. "When your internal metronome slows, you get a variety of benefits," says Mehmet C. Oz, M.D., director of the Heart Institute at Columbia University.

"You also lessen the risk of catastrophic events like heart attacks and strokes."[9] Everything from Parkinson's disease to various nervous system disorders, sleep disorders, neurological injury, learning disabilities, and psychological disorders have been treated through the therapeutic use of sound. The silent repetition of a mantra did not have the same benefits as chanting it out loud. According to the ancient Kundalini science of *Shabd Guru* (sounds that teach), when the tongue strikes the upper palate of the mouth, the reflex points there are being stimulated, which activates the nearby pituitary and hypothalamus by nonphysical energy channels that are similar to acupuncture meridians.

The American-based Kundalini Research Institute has documented the effects of mantra chanting on endocrinological stimulation. "Their research indicates," says Khalsa, "that the technology of the *Shabd Guru* has enabled people to recover from a wide range of conditions, including addiction to drugs and alcohol, depression, anxiety, chronic fatigue, neurosis, and sexual dysfunction."[10]

Long-Term Effects of Yoga

If Susan experiences these benefits at the beginning of her practice, what about the psychological effects on a person who has been practicing for many years? After a time of practicing Yoga regularly, says Khalsa, "you get a crossover from short-term to long-term biochemical changes. The long-term effect is the buildup of the changes you're producing daily."

David, a sixty-four-year-old pediatrician in Vermont with a long history of dysthymia, has had an on-again, off-again Yoga and meditation practice since he backpacked through India in the sixties. Nine years ago, he sold his medical practice so that he could write full-time. When, instead of writing four hours every day as he'd intended, he spent far too much time with the bells and whistles of his new computer, ordering special editing programs and how-to books, he became depressed at his lack of progress. Since he'd been practicing Yoga irregularly for years, he decided to take a month-long teacher training course, not so that he could teach, but to deepen and help him focus on his practice. During the course, he felt better than he had in years and committed to practicing every day. And in the nine years since then, he has written a novel and a children's book, which he self-published. He writes every day and volunteers in the county jail, teaching Yoga and meditation to prisoners. "I feel like I woke up to the true possibilities of my life when I turned fifty-five and began a daily practice," he says. "My practice keeps me centered and aware of my feelings, so that when bad things happen— and you can pretty much count on that after fifty—I no longer react by falling into a depression."

So far, most of the long-term studies that follow practitioners for several years have been done in the area of mindfulness-based training, the most recent of which was a large, controlled, three-country study published in the *Journal of Consulting and Clinical Psychology* (2000). The researchers used the Stress Reduction and Relaxation Program (SR&RP), developed by Jon Kabat-Zinn, Ph.D., at the University of Massachusetts, which includes Yoga stretches and postures, though the primary emphasis of the program is on mindfulness, a meditation technique where the practitioner observes his or her own mental process. We'll talk about this technique in greater detail in Chapter Eight. In the last twenty years, hundreds of studies at the University of Massachusetts, duplicated elsewhere, have shown a significant long-term reduction in anxiety and depression among participants who have taken the SR&RP. In the recent long-term study, SR&RP was combined with group cognitive therapy (a system that addresses our negative thoughts, which, it is assumed by this system, are the basis of our bad feelings about ourselves) as an eight-week treatment in the prevention of recurrence of major depression. In follow-up testing conducted a year later, the treatment group had a significantly lower relapse rate than did the control group. In language similar to what students might hear in a Yoga class, the study's authors say that the treatment encourages participants to "intentionally face and move into difficulties and discomfort, and to develop a decentered perspective on thoughts and feelings, in which these are viewed as events in the mind."[11]

That "decentered perspective" is what in Yoga we refer to as the development of Witness Consciousness. In the *Yoga Sutras*, Patanjali writes often of the "Seer." As the Seer develops through your practice, you begin to witness the circumstances of your life and the thoughts and feelings those circumstances engender with a calm, equanimous mind. This doesn't mean that we don't fully experience our feelings or that we ignore our thoughts. In fact, we may respond with more feeling than we did when we were depressed, especially if our depression was characterized by numbness. But the key word here is "respond," and we do so with equanimity and awareness, which Stephen Cope, in *Yoga and the Quest for the True Self,* calls the two pillars of Yogic practice.[12] Instead of feeling the compulsion to react, the practice of Yoga enables us to slow down the impulsive reaction and more calmly respond.

Though there have been numerous studies on the effects of Yoga practices on physical and emotional well-being in India, only a handful of studies have been done on Hatha Yoga in the West. And among these, there is a confusion of terms. In this book, I am using the word "Yoga" to mean "Hatha Yoga," the physical practice of postures that also includes breathing exercises and meditation. But in some Yoga studies, "Yoga" means only postures. In others it includes not only Yogic breathing and meditation, but also Yogic philosophy and attention to an ethical code. And then there are the variables such as the training and skill of the Yoga instructor, the environment the instructor creates in the class—is it accepting of how the practitioner is showing up on his mat right now, or is the emphasis on perfecting the posture?—and the frequency and duration of the class. But despite these discrepancies and variables and the sometimes less than scientific protocol, the indication is that Yoga, when practiced regularly (three or more times a week) in a session that includes simple breath awareness, can make a significant difference in emotional well-being. According to one study, Yoga does this physiologically by "relaxing chronic muscle tension and reducing unnecessary muscle activity, restoring natural diaphragmatic breathing, improving oxygen absorption and carbon dioxide elimination (which facilitates concentration and respiratory control), increasing alpha wave activity, and regulating the hypothalamus at an optimal level." A considerable list of benefits! "All of these factors," say the authors of a review of the literature on yoga and psychotherapy, "directly impact the autonomic and the central nervous systems, giving a logical explanation for the improvement of symptoms through Yoga."[13]

Vivekananda Kendra Yoga Research Foundation in Bangalore, India, and the National Institute of Mental Health and Neuroscience in India conduct ongoing research on the effects of mantra meditation, pranayama, and Yoga postures in a wide range of populations. In addition to the relaxation effect documented in studies throughout the world, the studies done in India show improvement in memory, cognitive functioning,[14] perceptual-motor skills,[15] muscle power, and visual perception,[16] indicating that Yoga practitioners are more alert and able to focus than are control groups who either exercised or did not alter their physical routine.

Another recent study in Bombay actually compared the effects of a Yoga practice done without meditation with the effects of a Yoga practice done with conscious breathing and meditation. In the study, "psychoneurotic patients" who had not previously responded to treatment were randomly divided into two groups matched for age, sex, diagnosis, and duration of illness. The patients were measured before and after six weeks of practicing Yoga five days a week. The Yoga-only group showed a significant improvement of 42 percent on standard assessment tools such as the MMPI, Rorschach, and Taylor Manifest Anxiety Scale. But the Yoga and meditation group showed a 73 percent improvement![17]

The authors of most of the studies conducted in India understood the importance of daily or regular practice. Unfortunately, some of the testing done in the United States lacks this understanding. For example, a six-month study that compared a once-a-week hour of group psychodynamic psychotherapy with a once-a-week hour of Yoga in the treatment of drug addiction showed far less impressive results. Both groups revealed mild positive correlations with reduced drug use, with no significant difference between them. Studies like these, when compared to the results of studies done in India, where Yoga practice was more frequent, underscore the need for regular, if not daily, practice.

Other studies have shown that when Yoga practice is more regular, there is a more significant improvement in depression, anxiety, and obsessive-compulsive disorder (OCD). One small study showed significant symptom reduction in patients suffering from OCD over the course of a year. Patients practiced one hour a day of Kundalini Yoga exercises that included specific pranayamas designed to stimulate the right side of the brain, often impaired in patients with OCD.[18]

One author hypothesizes that Yoga may be especially effective in treating seasonal affective disorder (SAD).[19] It is theorized that sunlight stimulates the pineal gland in the brain, which activates certain body chemistry. In the winter, when there is little sunlight directed toward the pineal gland, a seasonal depression, with all the symptoms of dysthymia, can set in. Yogic practices that focus the energy on the crown of the head, through inverted postures, special breathing exercises, visualizations, or by sounding certain tones, can directly stimulate the pineal gland. This stimulation, much like the success of phototherapy (special light that duplicates the sun's effect on the pineal gland), can activate the body chemistry to ameliorate SAD.

The specific techniques that may be used in a Yoga class—postures, pranayama breathing, meditation, toning, and relaxation—have all been shown, independently and together, to create an immediate biochemical state that feels good. However, more long-term, well-funded, controlled studies are needed before most doctors are willing to prescribe Yoga classes to their depressed patients. But practitioners like Susan and David aren't waiting for medical science to catch up.

Inversions

As we have seen, after a general session of Yoga that includes deep diaphragmatic breathing and stretching the body in all directions—side stretching, twists, forward bends, backbends, and inversions—you will feel better physically and emotionally. But let's look at a particular category of postures, inversions, to see more specifically how Yoga works to enhance mood and general well-being. Inversions refer to postures, like Shoulderstand, Headstand, and Handstand, in which the body is turned upside down.

Ann Brownstone, M.S., O.T.R., uses Yoga to work with those suffering from central nervous system disorders like multiple sclerosis and cerebral palsy, but has also found Yoga postures effective in treating anxiety disorder and depression. In her work with patients suffering from major depressive episodes, she has found that a full inversion like Headstand, done to the practitioner's tolerance level and with her assistance, has a positive effect on mood. According to Brownstone, one of the many therapeutic effects of an inverted posture is that it will increase tone and muscle extension in the postural muscles—neck, trunk, and limb girdle muscles responsible for erect carriage against the pull of gravity. In other words, the practice of inversions supports our standing posture—the spine is straighter and the head is in alignment with the spine—when we are upright. Mood is enhanced during and after inverted postures, Brownstone speculates, partly because an inversion challenges the sufferer's posture and muscle tone—think of the slumped shoulders of dysthymic depression. Our feelings show up in our posture, so addressing the "muscular" can have a profound effect on mood. In more scientific terms, Brownstone says that the increased extensor tone in the spine has a positive effect on the limbic cortex (emotional centers) and frontal cortical functioning in the brain.

There are enormous physiological benefits in the practice of inversions that lead to a general relaxation response. The gravitational stimulation of the carotid sinus, for example, causes the carotid sinus "to send messages to the medulla of the brain and cardiac centers that ultimately lower heart rate, respiration, and resting blood pressure."

Karen Koffler, M.D., director of Integrative Medicine at Evanston Northwestern Hospital, says that "inverted positions that are assumed in Yoga alter the blood flow (including lymphatic drainage) and flow of cerebral spinal fluid (CSF). If there is increased blood flow to the area, there will be increased bioavailability of oxygen and glucose—the two most important metabolic substrates for the brain. It follows then that cells bathed in a solution that is rich in factors required for the creation of neurotransmitters (like norepinephrine, dopamine, and serotonin) will be better able to produce these chemicals. In addition, altering the flow of CSF and, in fact, the compression of the caudal (or bottom) portion of the brain may itself improve overall brain function." This makes a lot of sense when you consider that the brain is maintained in a rather stagnant state all day, with the bottom portion constantly compressed. In fact, this is a component of craniosacral therapy, in which the therapist manipulates the skull and other areas of the body to improve CSF flow and improve function.

Based on her own experience and the experience of people she has taught, American Yoga College founder and director Rama Jyoti Vernon, who has been practicing Yoga for fifty years, feels that inversions can be beneficial for both anxiety and depression. She makes an important distinction, however: "Where we put the pressure on the head will determine the kind of mood shift we get." In her observation of thousands of students, she feels that pressure placed closer to the front of the head will lift a depressive attitude, whereas pressure on the crown stabilizes the mood and the emotions. A supported

Downward-Facing Dog Pose (*Adho Mukha Svanasana*) is an excellent posture that stimulates the front of the head and helps alleviate depression.[20] For pressure at the crown, Headstand (*Sirasana*) is an excellent posture. I do not recommend that you try this without instruction from a qualified teacher; however, you can find excellent guidance for entering, holding, and releasing the pose in *The Woman's Book of Yoga and Health*.[21] Because it activates the back brain, Vernon feels that Shoulderstand (*Sarvangasana*) is very calming. "It's a neutralizing pose, so whether there is depression or anxiety, it can be beneficial." It also stimulates the thyroid, so if the depression is related to hypothyroidism, Shoulderstand is especially useful.[22]

Inversions are generally done toward the end of Yoga practice. For obvious safety reasons, inversions should be learned from a qualified teacher who can teach you the safest way to enter, hold, and release an inversion without doing damage to your head, neck, shoulders, or back. People with unmedicated high blood pressure should not practice inversions. Yoga teacher and physiologist Roger Cole, Ph.D., suggests that there are conditions besides high blood pressure where inversions might be contraindicated. "These include congestive heart failure, elevated intracranial pressure, carotid artery stenosis (i.e., constriction), hiatal hernia (hernia in which part of the stomach protrudes through the esophageal opening of the diaphragm), stroke, neck problems, glaucoma (any of a group of eye diseases characterized by abnormally high intraocular fluid pressure, damaged optic disk, hardening of the eyeball, and partial to complete loss of vision), and detached retina."[23] In addition, inversions should not be practiced during menstruation, because you want your menses to flow out and down through your body, not back up toward the uterus.

Since it is vital that you learn to practice inverted postures from a qualified teacher, there are no instructions for inversions in this book. Because of their many therapeutic benefits for depression, you may want to discuss them with your teacher.

More Research Needed

It's vital that more research be funded to study the psychological effects of Yoga practice. Pharmaceutical companies carry out most of the research on depression. They are, with good reason, testing their own new medications. You won't find Eli-Lilly funding a study on Yoga. That is why government support in the evaluation of complementary medicine is so important. Unfortunately, when the White House Commission on Complementary and Alternative Medicine Policy (WHCCAMP) released its final report in March 2002, Yoga was not listed as a separate category under the "CAM Systems of Health Care, Therapies or Products." Nor is it shown under alternative systems (chiropractic, acupuncture, naturopathic, ayurveda, etc.) or mind-body interventions (meditation, hypnosis, guided imagery, etc.) or even somatic movement therapies (Feldenkrais, Alexander Method).[24] Instead, it was considered a kind of exercise or mentioned in relationship to meditation and relaxation techniques. Only through independent research, the publication of firsthand accounts—real people's stories like yours and mine—and educational efforts undertaken by organizations like the Yoga Research and Education Center (YREC), the International Association of Yoga Therapists (IAYT), and the Yoga Alliance will mainstream health care recognize what practitioners already understand—that Yoga is a powerful tool in the prevention and treatment of depression.

yoga experience

Before beginning a practice of postures, it's important that the muscles are gently flexed and stretched and that you exercise your joints to increase their mobility. Many Yoga books and videotapes suggest a series of specific warm-ups and joint-freeing exercises. In his book *Structural Yoga Therapy*, Mukunda Stiles recommends an excellent series that frees the joints and allows you to assess your mobility before beginning a practice. This series moves up the body, from the ankles to the neck and shoulders.[25] And there are wonderful warm-ups in *Kripalu Yoga: A Guide to Practice On and Off the Mat*.[26] Even a Yoga adept can sustain injuries if she has not taken the time to warm up her body.

It is not the purpose of this book to give you a complete sequence of postures to follow at home. It is important to begin your practice with a qualified teacher who can assess your body's needs. Many poses can be adapted for body type and ability. Here are simple warm-ups that provide a good stretch and flex for the spine. The spine is the house of the central nervous system, so maintaining flexibility in your spine is important for the health and vitality of all the systems of the body. Practice these simple exercises every morning, even if you don't have time for a complete Yoga practice.

Six Movements of the Spine

Cat/Cow (Spine Extension and Flexion)

These two movements for the spine contain the rudiments of both a backward bend and a forward bend. Come into a table position on your hands and knees, placing your palms directly under your shoulders and your knees beneath your hips, or a little wider for good stability.

Step One: As you inhale, lift your tailbone, then, vertebra by vertebra, lift your spine and look up through the crown of your head. In this

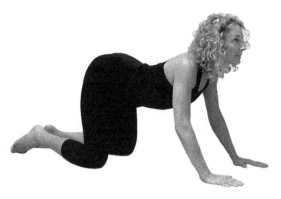

Cow: Inhale

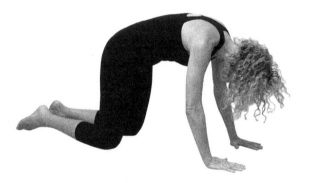

Cat: Exhale

position, your belly is like a hammock, stretching out of the house of your pelvis.

Step Two: As you exhale, round the spine like an angry cat, drawing your navel back toward your spine and your chin to your chest.

Slowly go back and forth between the two positions, undulating the spine and using deep breathing through the nostrils. Do this at least five times.

Side to Side

These two motions give a good lateral stretch to the spine. From the same table position, bring your right hip up toward your right ear, making a C curve with your body, like a human comma. Imagine you could put your right ear in your right hip pocket. Now move to the other side and do the same thing. Move back and forth slowly, from right to left,

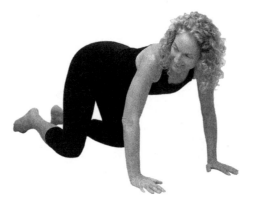

Side to side

exhaling through the mouth with a "ha" breath every time you move to the side and inhaling to center. Do both sides at least five times.

Threading the Needle

This is a wonderful stretch and twist for the spine. From table position, inhale your right arm up toward the ceiling, then exhale and bring that arm through the window of your left palm and knee and bring the right side of your head to the mat.

Continue to breathe deeply through your nostrils as you press your left fingertips into the mat to roll your left shoulder back for more of an upper-body twist. You can practice little micro-movements here, like moving the hips or rolling the head for a neck stretch. If you wish, you can lift your left arm into the air and explore various arm movements.

Enjoy the stretch for at least five long breaths through your nostrils. The body loves to twist. Play with it. Make it yours.

To come out of the pose, lower your left arm down and use it to press you back into table position.

Take a moment to close your eyes and unwind yourself. Trust the wisdom of your body to bring you back into balance. Then come back to a neutral table position and practice the same sequence on the other side. Enjoy. Make every movement count by paying attention to the breath and the sensations in your body as you practice.

When you return to table after threading the needle to the other side, again close your eyes and move in any way that brings you back into balance. Yoga is not about the "doing" but the "undoing" of all those tight places, the blocks in your body that trauma and loss have stored there. Imagine that you are dissolving another karmic knot (*samskara*) as you release. You probably are.

When you have completed the Six Movements for the Spine, come into Child Pose by bringing your buttocks back to your heels, resting your forehead on the mat, and drawing your arms alongside your body. If your buttocks aren't touching your heels, you may place a cushion between your hips and your heels for more support. It also feels good to bring a cushion underneath your forehead. Rest in Child Pose. Yoga is about balance. Take a moment to balance the "doing" of the Six Movements of the Spine with stillness. Relaaaaaax.

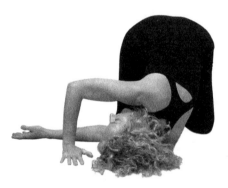

Threading the Needle: Exhale arm through

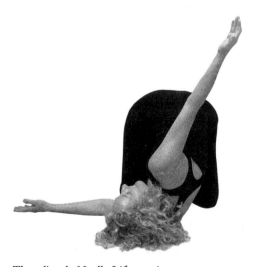

Threading the Needle: Lift opposite arm

fertilizing the ground— the healing principles of yoga

Yoga attempts to create a state in which we are always present—
really present—in every action, in every moment.

—T.K.V. DESIKACHAR, *The Heart of Yoga*[1]

Pouring the Foundation: Tapas, Svadhyaya Ishvara-pranidhana, Kriya Yoga

In Chapter One, we talked briefly about the Yoga system for positive mental health. Now, as you are beginning or deepening your practice, you may have more curiosity about the healing principles of that system. Your understanding alone won't cure your depression any more than just reading a self-help book will, but it will provide a foundation for your practice that will ease your recovery. As you begin to feel better, you may develop an enthusiastic curiosity about all aspects of the Yoga system.

In the first sutra in Chapter Two of *The Yoga Sutras*, Patanjali provides the foundation, a basic instruction for "union in action" (Kriya

Yoga). Union in action is daily life lived in a clear and conscious way—actions taken from an awakened state. This state, available to you always, is the blue sky beneath the weather of your current mood. Union in action rests on a sturdy tripod of willful practice (tapas), self-observation (svadhyaya), and surrender (Ishvrara-pranidhana). The strength of each leg of the tripod will support your recovery from depression. In my own recovery, it was necessary for me to cultivate all three. Practice alone would not have been enough. It certainly helped that I was willing to step onto my mat every day (tapas), but it was in doing so that I began to learn to listen to the messages my body was giving me (svadhyaya). Before I had a daily Yoga practice, I created a lot of discomfort for myself by *not* listening to my body. Sometimes I overate. Sometimes I drank too much alcohol. Sometimes I said "yes" when my body was saying "no." There were even times when I didn't acknowledge my body telling me it had to pee! What was going on in my head—the work I was doing or the meeting I was attending—was more important than my own body's signals. Also on my mat, I began to learn the lesson of surrender (Ishvara-pranidhana)—to take an action for its own sake and to allow myself to be totally absorbed in the effects, without expecting a particular outcome. As I learned the lesson of surrender on my mat, I had fewer expectations and demands of myself and others—and therefore fewer opportunities for disappointment.

Now, you don't have to know, identify with, or remember any of these Sanskrit words. If they irritate you, forget about them. It's the concepts that are important. First, we practice. The very act of stepping onto your mat is an act of *tapas*—willful practice. With disciplined practice, we light an inner fire that burns away our impurities. "Tapas" refers to both the willful practices (also called austerities) and the purifying inner fire that the practices produce. But practice alone will not support union in action and provide a full recovery from depression. As we practice, we also cultivate self-awareness. Here, the word *svadhyaya* is used, which means the study of self. In Classical Yoga, svadhyaya referred to the learning, by chanting, of the texts sacred to Yoga. This, it was believed, was the path to deeper self-knowledge. One form of self-study is the awareness you cultivate when you listen to your body as you practice.

But with only willful practice and self-study, we might become somewhat analytical and harsh—a kind of Yoga Nazi. So it's surrender, the third leg of our tripod, that softens the heart. And strengthens it, too. One of the hardest lessons to learn in life is when to let go—of a relationship, a dream, a fantasy, even a depression. Yet once we learn that we can't control people, things, and emotions, when we surrender to reality as it is, we are happier. *Ishvara-pranidhana* literally means surrender to the Lord, but Ishvara is a special kind of Lord, not one well known in the pantheon of Indian gods and goddesses. Rather, Ishvara comes closest to being the Lord of the transcendent Self, the self that is highest within you. It is your "personal" god. In the words of Swami Vivekananda, the great Vedanta sage who first brought the concepts of Yoga to the West when he appeared at the 1893 World's Parliament of Religions in Chicago, "Personal God is the reading of the Impersonal by the human mind."[2]

When you release from a posture after a long holding into a spontaneous flow of movements or into stillness, guided not by your mind but by your awakened energy, you are cultivating surrender to that "personal" God, your higher self.

Fires of Change: Tapas

The ancient Yogis believed that tapas, or inner fire, develops through the practice of self-discipline, or "austerities." For modern Yoga practitioners, this doesn't mean standing on one leg in the sun and rain for days on end. Rather, it is the self-discipline that brings you to the mat each morning to purify and strengthen your system through willfully held postures and breathing exercises that eliminate impurities in your body, your mind, and your emotions. Within this framework, says Viniyoga master Gary Kraftsow, "tapas is primarily the process of getting rid of something undesirable in our system—from chronic subliminal muscle contraction, to toxicity in the colon, to deep-rooted emotions and behaviors." With each session on your mat, you are building the strength to break through old patterns and past conditioning. With each session, you are strengthening your vital energy, or prana.

It's a threefold process. As your prana energy grows stronger, moving you out of depression, your self-awareness needs to grow, too. Prana, without a focused mind, is simply energy, and energy can easily be destructive. Violence is unleashed prana, unmodulated by the mind, or *chita*. When someone is in a manic state, there is too much prana in his system. Patanjali's formula—combining cleansing, energy-building practices (tapas) while developing a calm mind through self-study (svadhyaya), with the capacity to surrender (Ishvara-pranidhana)—is the key to positive mental health.

I know Yogis whose practice is so physical that they have burned away many impurities in their system and their prana is very strong. They burn with an intensity that is often physical, often charismatic. But, like David, a Yoga teacher and ski instructor in Colorado, the development of self-awareness has fallen behind. Years before he began a daily Yoga practice, David self-medicated with drugs and alcohol and, when he wasn't high, suffered from depression. Once he met his teacher, an Indian guru, he left his toxic life at a ski resort and joined his teacher's community in the mountains. In a way, Yoga became his drug. His practice was his addiction. He spent hours in his room, practicing postures and energizing pranayama breathing exercises. But he was not self-reflective, and he resisted meditation. His life, he said, was a meditation. What grew and strengthened in David was his prana energy, but it was untempered by self-awareness (svadhyaya). David was radiant from his practice and many people were attracted to him. His Yoga classes were popular, and he became sexually involved with a number of his students. David's high energy and low self-awareness got him into trouble so often that he was finally barred from teaching in his community. Prana must be strengthened in proportion with self-awareness, so that our actions come from a place of clarity.

Looking Inward: Svadhyaya

In ancient times, without the availability of books, knowledge was an oral transmission from teacher to student. As devotees chanted the sacred texts, committing them to memory, they were also gaining knowledge of the self. In the world of Yoga today, in addition to chanting, there are self-help books, workshops, and a wide variety of Yoga therapies—literally hundreds of ways to know the self. The way I know best is right on my Yoga mat—through self-observation. As your practice begins to burn

away the impurities, the obstacles to your freedom, you begin to cultivate a listening—to your body, to your mind, to your emotions. You can
cultivate this listening by observing your breath and the sensations in
your body as you practice. This takes intention and attention. It is easy
to practice Yoga as though it were exercise, moving from posture to posture, with little awareness of the sensations in your body or your feeling
state. This is unconscious Yoga, and though you will feel good afterward
and will receive many physiological and psychological benefits from
your practice, you run the risk of energetically reinforcing old patterns
and habits of mind.

When you practice Yoga with awareness of the sensations in your
body, your thoughts, and your feelings, you will grow in self-awareness.
And as you grow in self-awareness, you begin to have glimpses of what it
means to feel utterly and wholly connected, how your small self is not
separate from the Absolute, the Self of the universe. The moments of
awareness may be like slender threads that you follow as you release
from a Yoga posture or as you sit, observing your energy after a pranayama
breathing exercise. But as your practice deepens, the threads begin to
weave together, and you may begin to carry this awareness with you
off the mat—maybe for just a few minutes after your Yoga session,
maybe all day. Eventually, you may keep this awareness with you always.
You may become always aware of your wholeness. The cultivation of
self-awareness through your practice is an essential aspect, not only for
your recovery from depression but for the ultimate goal of your Yoga
practice—to become a *jivan mukti*, an awakened one. When you are
awake, there will still be pain in your life. Pain is inevitable, but you will
no longer suffer more as a result of your pain. You will remember that
beneath the temporary separation you may be feeling, you are whole.

Surrender: Ishvara-Pranidhana

Surrender is tricky. Does it mean giving up? Accepting defeat? Being
codependent? Letting the universe provide? Not in my book, and not in
the *Bhagavad Gita*, either. There, Lord Krishna tells the warrior Arjuna
that making plans, taking action, even painful action, is not only necessary but is the only way we fulfill our destiny (*dharma*). Where we get in

trouble is when we are attached to the fruits of our actions or our expectation of how things should be. Surrendering means working with what we've got, setting intentions and working toward them, but without attachment to the outcome.

Easier said than done. If you're organizing a party, you want people to come, and you might feel disappointed if only a handful of your friends helped you celebrate. But imagine how much more you might enjoy your small party if you said to yourself, "These are just the people who are supposed to be here. With fewer people, we can have more meaningful conversations and more intimate connections with one another." And whether you donate them to a soup kitchen or your neighbors, you can always think of something to do with the leftovers.

If you already have a felt sense of a relationship with the divine, Ishvara-pranidhana will be easy. The devotional practices, chanting the names of God, dancing, praying, will have an uplifting effect on your state of mind. On the other hand, an impediment to practicing Ishvara-pranidhana might be your uncertain relationship with the divine. What if you don't have one? For you, Ishvara-pranidhana may mean cultivating a state of openness, receptivity, humility, and gratitude. It may simply mean the practice of surrendering control over some aspect of your life, and trusting that if you can stay open and receptive, you will receive exactly what you need.

Yoga therapist and teacher in the Viniyoga tradition Leslie Kaminoff compares this important sutra about realizing union in action (*kriya-Yogah*) to the Serenity Prayer of Reinhold Niebuhr, used in the twelve-step recovery programs. Ishvara-pranidhana is about accepting that there are certain things in your life that are not within your control. "In order to know," he says, "when you're engaged in tapas [will] and when you're engaged in Ishvara-pranidhana [surrender], you need to know the difference between the two, which is svadhyaya [self-study]. The moment someone takes their first Yoga class, they are being asked to introspect about things they don't ordinarily introspect about. The process of introspection allows you to uncover the connections that are already there in your body." If you cultivate these three principles on the mat—willful practices that burn away the impurities, self-study, and surrender—your life will change.

Opening Your Inner Space: Dukha and Sukha

The word for suffering in Sanskrit is *dukha,* but it means much more than the English translation. The concept of dukha is bigger than suffering, bigger even than depression. The real meaning of dukha has within it the seeds of recovery from dukha. Literally, it means "obstructed space." Whenever there is depression, there is contraction. Some area of the body or mind is compressed; some area of the emotions is blocked. Depression, viewed this way, is treated by creating more space—*sukha*—which is exactly what you do when you practice Yoga. Yoga postures (asanas) and pranayama breathing exercises expand the lungs, decompress areas of tension, and release dammed-up emotions, creating a freer space within the body and mind. Most scholars translate sukha as "happiness," but the word literally means "unobstructed" or "open space." "Whenever someone comes to me," says Leslie Kaminoff, "whether it's for depression or a breathing difficulty or a back pain, what I'm assuming is that there is some place in the system that is obstructed, that needs more space. Whether the problem is in her joints, her spine, or with her breathing, there's a sense of congestion or blockage or obstruction." All the practices of Yoga—the asanas, the pranayamas, the chanting, and the meditations—address these blockages and begin to release them.

Loving Yourself

Practicing Yoga gives you the opportunity to do something loving for yourself. "Every single physical act triggers a change in your brain chemistry," Patricia Walden says, "so the more we do positive things like practicing Yoga, eating foods that are good for us, listening to inspiring music, reading poetry, seeing inspiring art, the better we feel." Every time you step onto your Yoga mat, if your intention is to listen to your body and honor your limitations, you are giving yourself the opportunity to practice self-love. In the eighties, I heard Yogi Amrit Desai, the then spiritual leader of Kripalu, say, "You can't really love somebody else without loving yourself. You can only extend to others what you have offered yourself." Beginning a Yoga practice, or practicing regularly if you've already begun, is the most generous way I know of loving yourself.

The kinds of messages you send to yourself, on and off your Yoga mat, make a difference in how you feel. When you give self-doubt and criticism free rein in your mind, you are setting yourself up for a felt experience of depression in your body and mind. Yoga can help you talk to yourself more gently. You are already practicing compassion toward yourself when you step onto your Yoga mat, and the self-accepting messages you send to yourself, even when you cannot fully come into a pose, go a long way in shifting the energy of depression. In Western psychotherapy, cognitive therapy has been shown to be especially useful in treating depression, because it seeks to reframe the negative thoughts you may have about yourself. For thousands of years, Yoga has addressed our thoughts and how we can reframe them, not only through physical practices that alter our perceptions and through the use of affirmations, which we'll discuss later in this chapter, but also through acceptance. The meditative techniques that we'll read about in Chapter Eight cultivate that sense of the acceptance of reality as it is. These techniques allow us to observe our thoughts, even sad or bitter thoughts, without judgment. This self-observation without judgment is the beginning of change. In addition, Yoga cultivates specific restraints (*yamas*) and observances (*niyamas*) that, for the sake of our emotional, mental, and physical well-being, provide guidance in our daily life.

Yogic Values: Yamas and Niyamas

We serve our own well-being and the well-being of others when we act in a way that is nonharming toward all beings, including ourselves. In the Yoga system, we can work with our actions through the cultivation of the *yamas* (restraints) and the *niyamas* (observances). The yamas and niyamas are the first two limbs of the Eight-Limbed Path suggested in Patanjali's *Yoga Sutras*. Since these guidelines for ethical behavior come before posture and breath and the other four limbs that address meditation, we can assume that Patanjali considered that living in alignment with these values was at least as important as the specific Yoga practices.

Who among us has not suffered when we feel that we've made a choice or fallen into a behavior at odds with our own values? Raoul Naroll, a cross-cultural anthropologist, emphasizes the importance of "moralnets," defined as "family and community connections that tie people together and provide an ethical background to what each individual does."[3] In other words, when faced with an ethical choice, your moralnet can provide the framework within which to make your decision. Research has shown that approximately 70 percent of the world's population lives in societies that have strong moralnets, where loyalty to a community overrides personal goals. That 70 percent doesn't include most of the Western world, which, according to ethicist and social philosopher Peter Singer, has been tending, "at least since the Protestant Reformation, away from community and towards a looser association of individuals."[4] Without connection to family, tribe, or community, the "moralnet" grows weak and the fabric of society is threatened by social breakdown and corruption. "Crime in America is the most vivid indication of the direction that a society of self-seeking individuals can take," argues Singer. "It is a frightening thought that we may be witnessing, in the United States today, the first large-scale society in which the moralnets have become too weak to support ethical ways of living."[5]

Moralnets can provide a sense of comfort. But they are hard to maintain in our mobile culture, where we change jobs, cities, and even relationships more often than the generations that preceded us did. Many of us have left the communities in which we were raised and abandoned the organized religions in which we were given a prescribed set of rules for choosing right from wrong. Without a moralnet, we feel isolated and alone. It is no wonder, then, that in Western society we are watching depression reach epidemic proportions.

Current research shows that though in hypothetical moral dilemmas we may make altruistic decisions for the good of all, in practical day-to-day moral decisions, even the simple injunction "do no harm" in the Hippocratic Oath is hard to live by when our own self-interest is at stake.[6] According to social psychologist Dennis Krebs, "The essence of morality lies in the idea that people have a duty to uphold the systems of cooperative exchange that have evolved in the groups to which they belong."[7] Certainly the success of the twelve-step recovery programs bears this out. The fellowship of Alcoholics Anonymous and the other recovery programs based on the AA model is in itself a moralnet, and the twelve steps are a formula for ethical behavior. Many people in recovery are more at ease with themselves, not only because they are no longer practicing their addiction but also because they have the comfort of the fellowship and the twelve steps to guide their choices.

The community of Yogins can also provide a moralnet, both in fellowship and in ethical guidelines. You don't have to live in an ashram or go on Yoga retreats to feel a part of a community of like-hearted people in a Yoga class. And whether you accept or ignore it, Yoga does provide a set of ethical guidelines in the yamas and niyamas. Let's take a look.

Yamas

1. *ahimsa:* nonharming
2. *satya:* truthfulness
3. *asteya:* nonstealing
4. *brahmacharya:* chastity
5. *aparigraha:* greedlessness

The first yama, or restraint, is *ahimsa,* or nonharming. This is the restraint that Gandhi practiced when he led Indians in nonviolent resistance to British rule. When we refrain from self-destructive activities like using drugs, smoking cigarettes, and other forms of addictive behaviors, we are practicing ahimsa toward ourselves, which is as important as practicing it in relationships with others. Violence arises out of fear and ignorance. As we grow in awareness, we become less fearful and our actions arise from understanding rather than ignorance. We naturally become nonharming in our actions.

As both a writing teacher and a Yoga teacher mentor supporting the development of new Yoga teachers, I have had the opportunity to see how my "critiquing" has changed over the years, moving from a style that may have occasionally caused harm to one that is more nonharming. As a professional writer and editor, I have often been hired to work with a manuscript to prepare it for potential publication. In the past, I approached a manuscript rather like a surgeon who looks only at the body part upon which she is about to operate. The effect of my words was occasionally harming to a writer's feelings about himself or his work. My intention was always to bring out the best in the manuscript, but in dealing only with the manuscript, and not with the feelings of the human being who wrote it, I was not practicing ahimsa.

As a Kripalu teacher mentor, I observe newly certified teachers and meet with them afterward to discuss the class. I know that the effect of my words can create an uplifting post–Yoga class meeting, where the new teacher feels empowered in her teaching and is open to receiving constructive comments for ways she might wish to change something about her class. In the mentoring process, I always begin with what I love about a teacher's approach. I tell her all the things she is doing right, how good it felt in my body to be led from posture A to posture B, and I repeat some of the wonderful things she said as she led the class. My role with the teacher is to help her grow into becoming the best teacher she can be, not according to my definition of what that might look like, but according to her own. I may need to share some points regarding her leading of a pose that adversely impacted the students' safety or some other aspect of their experience, but I do so in the context of the love I feel for all the things the teacher has done right. That is critiquing with ahimsa. And it is a practice I am still learning to develop in my work with writing students.

The second yama, *satya*, or truthfulness, is about practicing honesty, not only with others but also with ourselves. According to Kriya Yoga scholar and teacher Marshall Govindan, satya is not only about speaking the truth, it's also about sitting in silence. "So much of what is spoken is so unnecessary, so trivial and unreal. To cultivate silence, or to speak only what is edifying, after reflection, brings clarity to our minds and relationships."[8] When we lie, we are attempting to reshape reality in our own terms. When we are established in satya, we are able to accept reality as it is.

Patrick is a forty-two-year-old salesman who has been my Yoga student for several years. He is a kind and generous man, the kind of person who is always finding animals in need of care, always helping his friends. But he also exaggerates his accomplishments and sometimes even lies to impress others. Several times, I was aware that his grandiose stories about himself were skirting the edge of truth. When we worked together, designing a practice that would help him with his anxiety, he admitted that he often felt so anxious about the truth that he had to embellish it. Patrick grew up with an older sister who at an early age showed promise as a pianist, whereas Patrick considered himself tone deaf. This sister was also more athletic than Patrick and did better academically. It is not surprising that Patrick felt his sister received more love and attention from his parents than he did. As a young child, he began to make up stories or exaggerate the ones that were true, as a way of being noticed. Lying became a habit, and it was a problem in his adult relationships, particularly with women. It wasn't until Patrick began a daily Yoga practice that he started to develop an acceptance of himself as he was. Eventually, as he felt better about himself, the need to lie diminished. He told me that in cultivating truthfulness in his communications with others, he was feeling even better about himself, and that when he exaggerated, as he still did on occasion, usually when he was in an anxiety-producing social or work situation, he immediately regretted it. "If I lie now, instead of making me feel better, I feel like I've stepped out of my own truth, which is that I'm okay just the way I am."

The third yama, *asteya*, means nonstealing. It is obvious that taking from another darkens and constricts the spirit. If you must hide your actions or look over your shoulder, are you not obstructing your own spaciousness? You are probably causing yourself as much suffering (dukha) as your victim. But when you respect other people's boundaries, your own space is unobstructed, which, as I discussed above, is the definition of happiness (sukha). I have heard it said that feeling needy and greedy is a sign that some divine gift has been refused. If you acknowledge and are grateful for the gifts you have, the desire for more begins to dissolve.

The fourth yama, *brahmacharya*, or chastity, is perhaps the most complex. According to Classical Yoga, brahmacharya is defined as "the abstention from sexual activity, whether in deed, thought, or words."[9] Those on a path toward union with the divine may, even today, live as *sanyasins* (renunciates), maintaining complete sexual abstinence. However, in modern times, many Yogins have defined brahmacharya more simply as moderation in all sensual and sexual pleasures. Psychologists have long understood that what we deny and repress can be acted out in ways that are harmful to ourselves and others. For evidence, we have only to look at the many sex scandals that rocked the Yoga and Buddhist spiritual communities in the early nineties, involving gurus and their disciples, not to mention the uncovering of the problems in the Catholic Church in this decade.

For some, celibacy can open the door to a deeper intimacy with the divine. Their sexual energy may be channeled into devotion and service. But it's vital for the person who chooses total celibacy within the Yogic tradition to have done a thorough self-inquiry. When considering the total practice of brahmacharya, one must ask oneself: What am I avoiding? What am I afraid of? What am I running away from? What haven't I dealt with in my own relationships? Before walking the path of a renunciate, it is important to ask yourself if the very choice to abstain from a sexual relationship is a symptom of your depression. Are you attempting to prematurely transcend relationship? Is celibacy the path that will lead you to union with God, or are you avoiding true emotional and spiritual growth?

Most of us will not be choosing to practice brahmacharya in its most comprehensive form. Instead we can use the concept to examine our sexual behavior in and out of relationship. Are we using healthy restraint in our sexual impulses, or are we repressing them entirely—a kind of sexual anorexia—or are we indulging in sexual activities that may show a lack of compassion and love for ourselves and others? Brahmacharya for most of us may mean a variety of sexual experiences, practiced in the loving container of a healthy relationship. Art of Living founder Sri Sri Ravi Shankar defines brahmacharya as moving into Brahma or moving into infinity. In this context, the practice of brahmacharya may or may not include celibacy. Rather, brahmacharya is the increased strength one feels when "you see yourself as more than the body, as consciousness, as Brahman."10

The fifth yama is *aparigrahah,* or greedlessness. This yama teaches us that when we accumulate too many possessions, we become attached to them and fear their loss, a process that separates us from our true selves. That separation darkens our spirits and we feel depressed. Without the conscious practice of greedlessness, we may find that we make comparisons between others and ourselves. Accomplished as you may be in certain areas of your life, there will always be someone else who has skills or accomplishments or possessions you don't have. When you cultivate greedlessness, you are happy for your friend's success without feeling diminished by it.

Niyamas

1. *shauca:* purity
2. *samtosha:* contentment
3. *tapas:* austerity
4. *svadhyaya:* self-study
5. *Ishvara-pranidhana*: surrender to the Lord

In addition to the regular practice of the yamas, which, according to Yoga scholar Georg Feuerstein, helps Yogins moderate the "powerful survival instinct and rechannel it to serve a higher purpose,"[11] the second limb of Patanjali's Eight-Limbed Path are five practices or observances that address the Yogin's inner life, known as the niyamas. These include purity (*shauca*) of body and mind, and contentment (*samtosha*), which is being at peace with oneself and one's life exactly as it is in this moment, a practice that requires self-acceptance. Purity of body and mind and contentment are cultivated naturally in the practice of the next three niyamas—willful practice or austerity, self-study, and surrender. Yes, these are the same three observances that we discussed earlier in the chapter, when we were talking about Yoga on the mat. Here, though, Patanjali is suggesting that we cultivate these three aspects— tapas, svadhyaya, and Ishvara-pranidhana—off the mat as well. As tapas is used here, it means austerity. In modern terms, for those of us in the everyday world of commerce, simply cultivating a regular Hatha Yoga practice may be considered an austerity. When you willfully bring yourself to your mat each day, you are making a commitment to burn away the impurities in your system, including your depressive symptoms. In your everyday life, tapas may also mean forgoing pleasure-seeking activities that dull the senses and numb the mind.

Svadhyaya, the fourth niyama, which, as we've already seen, Patanjali considered essential for achieving the union in action that is Yoga, refers to study, the purpose of which is not more information or even intellectual learning. Rather, it is a knowing of the true nature of self. This knowing of self unites us with Self or God. In other words, our study— whether through reading and chanting of scriptures; listening to inspiring teachers; observing the sensations, thoughts, and feelings that arise in a Yoga posture; dreamwork; or meditation in which we observe the self—leads us to the understanding that we are not separate from God or ourselves. Therapy, too, can be a form of svadhyaya if it penetrates beneath your symptoms, your stories, and the system of neurotic complexes and defenses you've constructed to survive your childhood to uncover your divine nature. Even if you don't believe that your nature is divine, even if you are an atheist, the observation of self, without judgment, will allow you to live from that clear place of union in action that is Yoga.

The fifth niyama is surrender to the Lord (*Ishvara-pranidhana*). We discussed this important aspect of Yoga in action on pages 78–79. It is in the practice of surrender that all separations disappear. In relationships, cultivating the capacity to surrender, whether in an argument across the dining room table or in lovemaking, allows you to be more fully present to your experience with your partner. In this context, Ishvara-pranidhana can mean that separations between you and your partner may begin to dissolve so that you experience the wholeness of sacred union with the divine through your partner.

On the way to such a union, the very acts of devotion—whether to your partner in the form of openhearted giving, or to the divine in the form of praying and chanting—can lift the spirit out of depression. Here's a mantra I use when I practice that cultivates the acceptance of, and surrender to, reality as it is: "Thy will be done, not mine." (*Om namo bhagavate Vasudevaya.*)

Often, as I hold a pose, I use a mantra along with my breath to cultivate my own sense of surrender in the posture. Sometimes I will repeat the mantra "Thou art with me," but I do so with a personal awareness that there is no separate "Thou"—that, in fact, *I* am that "Thou," and that *you* are that "Thou." There is no separation from the energy of the divine. "You are that" (*Tat tvam asi*) is a traditional mantra from the Advaita Vedanta tradition of nondualism that tries to express in words the inexpressible concept of this wholeness. "*Tat tvam asi,*" I say, again and again, and I repeat the words, "Thou art with me." When I release, I feel an expanding sense of contentment (samtosha), and I believe that in holding and releasing, again and again, I am purifying (shauca) my body and mind.

These restraints and observances are in themselves a program for positive mental health, but, when studied together with the specific breathing practices that constitute the pranayamas, the postures that constitute the asanas, and the meditation practices, they form a system for maintaining a full life free from depression.

Accentuate the Positive

"When bound by negative thoughts," says Patanjali, "opposite ones should be cultivated."[12] Many interpreters understand this sutra as a conscious effort to think positively through the use of affirmations. The placement of this sutra just after a discussion of the yamas and niyamas, the first two limbs of the Eight-Limbed Path, seems to indicate how influential the ancient Yogis considered our thoughts in affecting our moods. This sutra suggests that we have the power to change our thoughts and thereby cultivate a sense of well-being. In many Hatha Yoga traditions, affirmations, or positive statements we make to ourselves, are the way we can work with our thoughts.

When we feel emotionally wounded, affirmations, along with postures, pranayamas, and visualizations, can speed the healing process. "Emotions," says Lisa Powers, an Ananda Yoga teacher, "are patterns of energy. When energy patterns get reinforced, over time they become very strong and difficult to dislodge or even recognize." Since Yoga works directly with energy, when we practice regularly, we have the opportunity of "creating strong new patterns of positive energy."[13] On her videotape, "Yoga for Emotional Healing," Lisa suggests that the first step in changing those patterns is to completely relax the body. "Tension is a result of blockages in our energy flow caused by emotional reactions to life."[14] When we can begin to release the tension in the body through our practices, we can more easily be guided by the underlying energy of the universe. If, as we've discussed, suffering is obstructed space, then it makes sense that when you begin to relax and dissolve those obstructions, you are more in the flow of life.

Think of a moment when you were happy. Try to imagine the scene in your mind. Chances are, it was a time when you were totally absorbed in your actions and your mind was one-pointed and focused. Perhaps you were singing or writing or swimming or running or making love or floating on a raft in the sun. You were in the flow.

When your body is beginning to relax on your mat, and your mind is absorbed in the breath or the details of a posture, you are in the flow and your mind is more receptive to change, to moving beyond your fixed ideas about your own limitations. Introducing an affirmation at such a moment can help facilitate that change. Affirmations can be practiced while holding a posture, releasing a posture, or in a resting position. For example, while standing in Eagle Pose, which involves twisting and balancing the body at the same time, Lisa Powers suggests the affirmation "In the center of life's storms, I stand serene."[15] When faced with a difficult situation that engenders fear, you might want to experiment with the affirmation "I live protected by the infinite light. So long as I live in the heart of it, nothing and no one can harm me."[16]

Does telling yourself that you live in the heart of infinite light make it so? Not exactly. We live in a world where suffering exists, where "bad things happen to good people," where, in fact, there may be times when we feel too depressed to stand in the light, to do the practices we know from past experience will make us feel better. Affirmations may not work if, deep down inside, you do not believe them. "The Yogis believe that we have to first make changes at the subconscious level for them to become operative in our conscious life," says founder of the American College of Yoga Rama Jyoti Vernon.

In fact, if I tell you that there is something that lies beneath your present sorrow that is always happy, you may feel worse because on a subconscious level you don't believe it's true. Striving for happiness by using simplistic affirmations that don't address your core belief system may be doomed to failure. We may be able to temporarily manipulate our mood with our affirmations to create a happy, even blissed-out state of mind, but it is likely to be a premature transcendence. If the affirmation is not grounded in our subconscious belief system, an hour later those negative thoughts may assert themselves again. "Positive thinking," says Sri Sri Ravi Shankar, "can even be a source of depression. The more you try to force that positive thought, the negative thought goes deep somewhere inside you."[17]

However, when affirmations are built on the foundation of your own belief system, they can begin to effect change at the level of the subconscious. Once again, even in designing affirmations for ourselves, it's important to meet our preconceived notions where we are. Confronting a belief with its opposite probably won't work. For example, the poet and essayist Lucy Grealy, whose 1994 memoir *Autobiography of a Face* was, according to *The New York Times*, a "contribution to the literature of the self," could not confront the belief that she was ugly by telling herself she was beautiful. When she was nine, she had a virulent form of cancer that destroyed her jaw and severely disfigured her face. Despite numerous operations, the structure of her face was never returned to her. Lucy believed she had an ugly face. You could not tell her she was beautiful, because she wasn't. But she was lean and spry and beautiful when she danced. Her mind was elegant, her wit was wry, and the beauty of her spirit soared on the written page. Lucy was only thirty-nine when she died at the end of 2002 of a drug overdose.

I knew Lucy at the Bennington College Writing Seminars, where I received a master's degree in writing and literature and she taught creative nonfiction. I can't say whether Yoga might have made a difference in Lucy's life. Perhaps it's some form of hubris on my part to wish that she had been in my class. I wish I had had the opportunity to ask Lucy to close her eyes and dive beneath her physical body, her emotional body, home to the ground of her being, where she was whole and beautiful. It might not have saved her life, but I wish I had told her how beautiful she was beneath her ravaged face. She might have dismissed my compliment if I'd said it in a classroom or over lunch, or even on the dance floor. But if she were in the flow, mind absorbed, body relaxed, awake to her energy in a Yoga pose, for that moment, on her Yoga mat, she might have believed me.

Meeting Your Belief

Rami Katz, a Kundalini Yoga teacher and therapist, makes a point to work with her client's belief system, using affirmations she cocreates with her client to support a shift in the client's distorted thoughts about herself. In Rami's opinion, the best use of affirmations is not mindlessly repeating a generic affirmation about living in infinite light, but something that is specific to the client's own ethos.

"For someone who is dysthymic," Rami notes, "we're often working with a belief system that pulls the person down—'not good enough,' or 'not okay.'" For example, one patient told her he was upset with himself because he was not consistent. Rather than a true inconsistency in his character or actions, what Rami saw was the client's perfectionism. Though Rami might agree with her client that there may be certain aspects of his personality that seem to him to be inconsistent, and he may be inconsistent in certain areas of his life, she reminded him of the consistency of the energy flowing through him. With Rami's help, the client was able to create his own affirmation: "Consistency breathes through me."

What Rami has found in her work with clients is that it's important to coordinate the self-created mantra or affirmation with the breath and with movement. "Though breathing alone can make someone feel better physically, they can easily relapse into the depressed feeling because the mind goes back to its old beliefs. When the mind is focused along with the breath, it works much better than just breathing." By giving both the mind and body tasks—an affirmation together with a simple repetitive movement and the breath—it is easier to reframe the negative belief.

In Yoga class, with students who are receptive to mantra chanting, Rami will use traditional Kundalini mantras to help them focus. With clients who have a strong religious belief system, Rami will work with that system. She's suggested everything from "Jesus loves me" to the use of "Hashem" for an Orthodox Jewish client. "When I worked with a Navajo woman, I said, 'Okay, give me a word that you would use when you're feeling insecure and are calling out for support from a higher power.'" Whatever mantra or affirmation Rami creates with her client, it is always coordinated with the breath. For Rami, meeting the client where he is, designing an affirmation that meets and challenges his negative belief system, works much better than imposing an affirmation or mantra.

Creating your own affirmation is great. Start with a phrase that is not in conflict with your belief system. Lucy Grealy would never have been able to believe an affirmation like "My face is beautiful," but perhaps, if she were using an affirmation like "Beauty breathes through me," along with other purifying Hatha Yoga practices, she might have begun to see the beauty in her life.

Language

Some teachers talk only about the physical body in a Yoga class—the placement of the feet, the alignment of the spine, and so on. That may suit you fine, and as long as you are breathing consciously and the sequence of poses is complete with forward and back bends, side stretches, twists, and inversions, you will begin to feel better. But your recovery may be hastened by language in your Yoga class that speaks to the unconscious. Many teachers feel that the language used in class can have a direct effect on their students' experience of releasing and going deeper in a pose. You may wish to find a teacher—and he or she can come from any tradition—who uses language that speaks to your heart.

Metaphors can speak directly to the physical and emotional bodies, circumventing the analytical mind. What would it be like to ease into a posture and, as international Yoga teacher Angela Farmer describes, to slither like a serpent, letting the inner body—the belly, the kidneys, the vital organs—initiate the movement? Or as Farmer's partner, Victor Van Kooten, says, to "move like a snail emerging from its shell, carrying the outer body along"?[18] Julia Mines, a Kripalu Yoga teacher, watches her students' response to her language while they are holding a posture. "I observed that as students lengthened or twisted to 'this body is a good one, this body is worthy of your love,' they responded the way a flower turns toward the sunlight for sustenance."[19] These instructors and others believe that visual metaphors transcend the conscious mind and speak directly to the body.

There is one metaphor that arises from the most ancient traditions of Hatha Yoga, and it supersedes all others: *Your body is a temple of the divine.* Years ago, when I did my first teacher training at Kripalu Center, we often began with a *sadhana* (practice) prayer that reminded us of this sacred knowledge. I share it with you now so that, if you wish, you may use it as an invocation before you begin your Yoga Experience.

> I open my heart to explore the divinity inherent within my body.
> I recognize that my body is the temple of the divine,
> and I am not just this body but the embodied spirit itself.
> During this sadhana time, my intention is to be present
> in my body and in the light of consciousness.

Whether or not you embrace the healing principles outlined in this chapter, whether or not you are able to envision your own body as "the temple of the divine," your body, mind, and spirit will come into balance through the everyday practice of Yoga, including pranayama breathing and meditation, and your depression will lift.

yoga experience

Here's a simple practice that both soothes and energizes, so it's wonderful to do when you're feeling anxious, and it lifts the depressed mood as well. This practice combines a special breath with a posture and an affirmation.

Part I — Breath to Fortify the Nerves

Come into a standing position with your feet parallel and one fist's width apart for stability. Draw your tailbone down. Lift your shoulders up to your ears, take in a breath, make fists of your hands, tighten the muscles of your face, hold the breath. Squeeze all the tension into a little ball at the back of your neck. Hold, hold, hold, for as long as you can. Then release the breath through your mouth, sighing out the tension, the "to do"s, the obsessive little thoughts, the expectations for how you're supposed to show up. They're not serving you. Let them go.

Pause and notice where you are feeling open and relaxed. Notice where there may still be tension and discomfort in your body.

Now stretch your arms out in front of your waist, palms face up. Inhale and make fists of your hands. While holding the breath, pump your fists back toward your waist. Exhale and relax. Close your eyes and feel the effects of the breathing exercise. Repeat.

Part II — Mountain Pose (Tadasana)

Stand with your eyes closed, your arms by your sides, and your palms turned out. Feel the energy you've generated in the breathing exercise circulating through your body. Notice the tingling in your arms and down into your hands. Feel the energy pulsing in your palms. Ground into the four corners of your feet and make sure they are parallel, either big toes touching or a couple of inches apart for more stability. Engage the muscles of the legs, thighs, and those around the knees, without locking the knees. Press the tailbone toward the ground, leveling the pelvis. Lift your torso out of your waist and draw your shoulders down and back. Slowly begin to lift your arms out to your sides as though you are making an offering of this energy. Bring your arms over your head with the palms facing each other. Relax your shoulders down again. Continue breathing slowly and deeply through the nostrils, filling with life breath—prana. Feel as though you are holding your arms up, not from your shoulders, but from the core of your body. Ground your feet and experience your connection to the earth. Feel the energy pulsing between your hands. Focus on your breath. Allow your breath to fill this vessel you've been given for this lifetime with life energy, strengthening this vessel so that you can hold more prana, more light, more joy; expanding your chest, your heart, your lungs, so that there's more room inside for your authentic expression of self. Hold this position for at least ten long breaths.

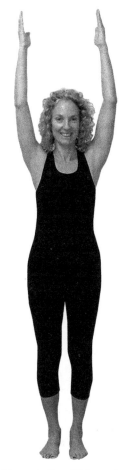

Mountain Pose (Tadasana)

Part III—Affirmation

Continue to hold Mountain Pose and breathe deeply through the nostrils. Relax into the sensation that's strong in your body. Bring the breath there. Bring the attention there and dive through that window of sensation into a deeper experience of being in your physical body in this moment, in Yoga, in union.

Now affirm to yourself: "I am aligned with the energy of the universe, and the energy of the universe supports and protects me." However, if this affirmation feels uncomfortable in any way, don't use it. Try an affirmation you can believe. How about "I am the energy I feel" or "I am aligned with my highest good?"

When you feel complete, slowly release the pose, lowering your arms to your sides. Stand with your feet a comfortable distance apart, your eyes closed, and your arms at your sides, palms face out. Breathe. Relax. Feel. Watch. Allow. You are energy!

lotus of many petals— the ways we practice

This being human is a guest house.
Every morning a new arrival.
A joy, a depression, a meanness,
some momentary awareness comes
as an unexpected visitor.
Welcome and entertain them all!

—RUMI, from "The Guest House"[1]

Your Yoga Practice

Whether the class you have enrolled in is called White Lotus, Bikram, Iyengar, Ashtanga, Kripalu, Integral, Sivananda, Svaroopa, Jivamukti, Anusara, or any of the other schools of Yoga, you are practicing Hatha Yoga, and you are already choosing positive mental health. Your decision to practice Yoga emerges from your own reservoir of mental health—your own inner wisdom—particularly if, in this moment, you are suffering. Take a moment to honor and acknowledge yourself.

The many types of Yoga mentioned above are all forms of Hatha Yoga. The word *Hatha* literally means physical force. Hatha Yoga is a practical physical system for aligning body, mind, and spirit, enhancing a sense of well-being, and managing and perhaps even eradicating your depression. While it is a system practiced by some but not all Hindus, Jews, Christians, Moslems, atheists, and agnostics also practice it. A young woman I know, who is a religious Jew, understands the importance of aligning and relaxing her body and mind and organizes Yoga classes with other Orthodox women.

No matter what form of Hatha Yoga practice you try—I'll describe some schools here in relation to depression and more in Chapter Ten—there are four important rules:

1. Breathe!

Unless instructed otherwise by a qualified Yoga teacher, always breathe deeply and slowly through the nostrils while entering, holding, and releasing a pose. The postures themselves are not magic positions; it is your breathing that gives them the power to heal. In some cases, if you're not breathing deeply and slowly, it is even possible to make your situation worse. Sally, a Rhode Island Yoga teacher, says that back in the seventies when she first took Yoga classes, her teacher did not talk about the breath, resulting, she believes, in the exacerbation of a misaligned rotation in her hipbone that has caused compression in her sacrum since birth. While Sally's lifelong tendency toward depression is endogenous, which means it has no known origin, she believes it is the compression in her sacrum that may be responsible for her depressive symptoms. If you are not conscious of your breathing in your Yoga practice, the practice may not help you manage or eliminate your depression. In fact, it might, as Sally believes happened to her, make it worse.

2. Listen to Your Body

Let your body be your first teacher. If you are paying attention to the sensations you feel as you practice, you will know when to release a pose or modify it. Yoga is not a competitive sport. Practicing with others in a class does not make you a member of a synchronized Yoga team. You are an individual with a different body, a different set of life experiences, injuries, and abilities than the twenty-something or the sixty-something practicing next to you. You can hurt yourself in Yoga if you push or strain or forget to breathe. Relax into the pose by breathing deeply, using micromovements to move in and out of your body's full expression of the pose. Listen to the sensations you feel and moderate your pose to accommodate them.

3. Sequence Your Poses

Each pose you practice has a stimulating or soothing effect on the chakras and the glands in your body. For example, the thymus gland is stimulated in backbending poses, which strengthens your immune system. It's important to practice a sequence that balances the energy in the chakras and glands. This means following a basic routine established by a qualified Yoga teacher. Unless contraindicated because of a medical condition from which you suffer, your Yoga session should include backbends, side stretching, twists, forward bends, and inversions.

4. Learn the Locks from a Qualified Teacher

The locks (*bandhas*) are three internal lifts that make your practice of postures and pranayamas more powerful and should be learned from and practiced with a qualified teacher, not from a book. On the other hand, they are so intrinsic to Yoga that you may find your body naturally lifting up internally as you practice. You may find that in certain standing poses you are naturally drawn to lift the pelvic floor. This is a simulation of the root lock (*mula bandha*), and it protects the lower back, particularly in backbends. It also gives you strength in standing postures. You will find that the abdomen naturally draws back toward the spine in certain postures, particularly in forward bends and in some breathing exercises. This motion simulates the stomach lock (*uddiyana bandha*). *Uddiyana* literally means "to fly up." When you draw the abdominal organs up and in, you are creating a natural upward flow of energy. In other postures, like Shoulderstand and Forward-Bending Head-to-Knee Pose, your chest will naturally lift to meet your chin. This simulates the throat lock (*jalandhara bandha*), and it compresses and stimulates the thyroid gland. When the locks occur spontaneously in a pose, don't resist them. But do not consciously practice them without first receiving guidance from a qualified Yoga teacher.

Schools of Hatha Yoga

There are numerous systems and schools of Hatha Yoga, all of which base their practices on the tripod we talked about in the last chapter— willful practice (tapas), self-study (svadhyaya), and surrender (Ishvara-pranidhana). Some traditions create Yoga in action (*kriya-Yogah*) through the doorway of the physical body, first cultivating willful practice (tapas). Other traditions enter through the doorway of inquiry or self-study (svadhyaya), while other traditions step through the doorway of the emotional body or surrender (Ishvara-pranidhana). If you have a committed practice, no matter which doorway you enter, you will come to the same place—the balance of tapas, svadhyaya, and Ishvara-pranidhana that is complete union. All Yoga traditions aim for a healthy body and a balanced mind, unobstructed by tension. Systems that enter through the doorway of the physical aspects of the practice (tapas), like Iyengar, the Vinyasa flow styles, or Bikram Yoga, have the potential to heal depression, not only through the physiological benefits discussed in Chapter Three, but also by distracting the mind from its negative self-talk.

Most people, when they sign up for their first class, don't make a distinction between the schools of Yoga. If asked, a new student will likely say he "thinks" he's practicing Hatha Yoga, and, of course, he is, because Hatha encompasses all forms of physical practice. So why make a distinction? It's my opinion that certain personality types are more comfortable beginning with a physical approach, while other people suffering from depression respond better to an approach that consciously creates an emotional as well as a physical container of safety for the practitioner.

The Indian system of Ayurvedic medicine (Ayurveda) acknowledges these basic differences in our individual constitutions, too. Ayurveda, which literally means "the wisdom of life," identifies three personality/body types or constitutions (*doshas*), which are determined at conception but are influenced and modified by the environment in which we grow up and the changes we face on a daily basis. The *vata* constitution is usually thin, wiry, and leans more toward anxiety than depression. If you are vata, you might wish to begin vigorously, but you would likely benefit most from a calmer, slower, more grounding practice with a long relaxation at the end. The *pitta* constitution is more fiery, likely to have a florid complexion and a medium but sturdy build. Pitta folks are often barrel-chested and are prone to high blood pressure. If you have a pitta constitution, you will likely benefit from a relaxing, cooling practice. The *kapha* constitution is heavier and slower. If you are kapha, you might wish to begin slowly, becoming more vigorous near the end of your practice to counteract your tendency toward sluggishness. Can you see that even if you are not suffering from depression, you, as an individual constitutional type, may be more drawn to one form of practicing Yoga than another?

Yoga and Ayurveda make a further distinction in categorizing three basic psychological states, called *gunas,* that more closely align with dysthymia and anxiety-based depression. When seen through the double lens of Ayurveda and Yoga, dysthymia resembles the *tamasic* (inertia) state and anxiety-based depression is more *rajasic* (aggressive). When we are feeling good, we are *sattvic* (balanced)—our rajas qualities are in harmony with our tamas qualities. I mention the Ayurvedic concepts here not to confuse you, but because the doshas and the gunas are terms you may encounter in your Yoga class. They are simply categories that give us another way to understand ourselves and to determine the kind of Yoga practice that may be just right. But if you're finding all these Sanskrit words and Ayurvedic terms confusing, stick to the basic understanding of your symptoms as described in Chapter Two.

Finally, there's another way to distinguish the kind of practice you might find most appropriate for you. If you are a person who is most comfortable with a linear and orderly approach to life—perhaps you favor mathematics and science and logical discourse—you may find that studying the B.K.S. Iyengar method, with its fine attention to the details of alignment, suits your personality. If you suffer from an anxiety-based depression, have been diagnosed with PTSD or a biochemical depression, you may wish to begin by placing the emphasis of your practice on purifying and bringing balance into your physical body (tapas)—balancing the endocrine system and stimulating the biochemistry of your brain. While all Yoga practices that include the requisite sequence of postures—side stretching, forward bending, backbending, twists, and inversions—will do this, in an Iyengar Yoga class you will work almost exclusively with the physical body to accomplish this, usually without reference to your emotional state.

The same is true in the Bikram sequence of poses and the flow Yoga sequences like Ashtanga and Power Yoga. If you are young and fit, the vigorous flow Yoga sequences may be particularly appealing. The anxious mind rests easy when it knows that the body will be taken through the same sequence of poses each time you come to the mat, which is the case with Bikram and the Vinyasa flow sequences, though not with Iyengar Yoga.

If, in your journey out of depression, you are interested in looking at what's true in your emotional body as you practice, you may be drawn to a Yoga tradition like Viniyoga, in which you begin with a self-inquiry: What does my body need today? Do I begin slowly with a restorative pose, moving into a more vigorous practice as my energy increases? Do I begin vigorously with sun salutations, to meet my already heightened energy? This is the doorway of self-study (svadhyaya). In a Viniyoga practice, the sequence of poses may vary, and breathing exercises are practiced that help you access and moderate your deeper feelings.

In Kripalu Yoga, the third doorway, the capacity to surrender (Ishvara-pranidhana) creaks open, even as the other two doorways, willful practice (tapas) and self-study (svadhyaya), are beginning to open. In this chapter, I'll share with you my own experience of a Kripalu Yoga session, and how it affects me, moment to moment, as I move through willful practice, self-study, and surrender. But first, let's look at some other schools of Yoga. Since I neither practice nor teach in these traditions, I have talked with senior teachers from these lineages who have helped their students recover from depression.

Iyengar Yoga—Aligning It All

Iyengar Yoga is a system developed by master teacher B.K.S. Iyengar, based on his studies with Krishnamacharya, the great Yoga Master of Hatha Yoga. B.K.S. Iyengar is credited with his innovative use of props to safely support students in poses, so that anyone of any size or any age or nearly any infirmity can benefit from Yoga. Many of the most well-respected Yoga teachers in the world have been or continue to be students of B.K.S. Iyengar. His strict and uncompromising approach to maintaining the purity of the practice of Hatha Yoga is the foundation from which a number of well-known teachers have developed their own systems. The doorway into an experience of Iyengar Yoga is through tapas, the purifying practices that build the inner fire. Without directly addressing the emotional body in the way some other systems do, Iyengar Yoga is a practice that soothes and calms the emotions through the physical practice of the postures. "The impact of yoga is never purely physical," says Iyengar. "Asanas, if correctly practiced, bridge the divide between the physical and mental spheres. Once we become sincere practitioners of yoga, we cease to be tormented by unhappy and discouraging states of mind."[2]

Australian Iyengar practitioner and teacher Christine Thompson feels that the focus involved in aligning the body into each posture helps her deal with her depression by changing her state of mind. "When I change my body position, it brings a change of attitude, my mind clears a little, and I can look at the problem more clearly." Rather than engaging the feelings directly, Iyengar Yoga works to heal the heart by refocusing the agitated mind on the specific alignment of the body in a pose. It is impossible to be obsessing about your problems when you are paying attention to the details of your alignment in Mountain Pose (*Tadasana*), one of the postures B.K.S. Iyengar recommends for depression. For example, he suggests that you "distribute your weight evenly on the inner and outer edges of your feet, and on your toes and heels. Tighten your kneecaps and open the back of each knee. Turn in the front of your thighs. Tighten your buttocks. Pull in your abdomen, and lift your chest."[3] With all these details and more to attend to, where is there room for your depressed thoughts? In his book *Yoga: The Path to Holistic Health*, Iyengar recommends a specific series of postures for depression, as well as sequences for many other conditions. In Chapter Two we talked about psychiatrist Janis Carter's work with patients suffering from PTSD. It is Iyengar's sequence for depression that produced such good results.

In his essay in the book *How We Live Our Yoga*, Boston-based filmmaker and writer Robert Perkins describes the six years he spent in "Yama-Yama land," the depression he entered after his wife died of breast cancer in 1994. Six months after she died, he says he had "ground to a halt. On the outside I didn't look any different, but I was a wreck. I couldn't sleep. My enthusiasm evaporated. I had no appetite. I drank too much. I ate a lot of Spam."[4] Desperate for relief, he began working privately with senior Iyengar Yoga instructor Karin Stephan, who, with Patricia Walden, opened the Boston Iyengar Center in 1985. Karin works privately with students in the Cambridge area and leads workshops on Yoga for depression in New York City and elsewhere. Karin doesn't impose a practice on her students, but rather, lets their bodies and their minds speak to her, using what she calls her "peripheral vision." She may be interacting with a student, listening to her speak, watching how she holds her body, how she moves it, and "all the while, I'm getting another message from the side of my mind, and that message is what I work with. It's like a ray of light that comes in at an angle from a window."

So when Robert Perkins showed up for his meetings, or didn't—for a year and half he "protected himself," sometimes scheduling private sessions, then not showing up—she intuitively knew to let the practice emerge. In his essay, Robert describes lying in the afternoon light that streamed in through Karin's west-facing windows. "I had no energy. I would lie in that light, softly crying. Occasionally, she would get me to work on my body a little."[5] Karin honored the bleakness of his sojourn in Yama-Yama land, never pushing him. Eventually she was able to get him to move, leading him in asanas that would stimulate his adrenal glands and kidneys and give him more energy. Together they did backbends and inversions. Slowly, Robert traveled back to a place where he was ready to engage with others.

Karin worked patiently, waiting for Robert's return. As a teacher, Karin is more interested in giving her students "a sense of their own capacity for change, rather than the change itself—something that has a ripple effect after they've seen me." In practical terms, this means that the practice she teaches to one person may be very different from the practice she teaches to another. But in general, for someone who exhibits the physical manifestations of dysthymia—the slumped shoulders, the shallow breath—she might work first with postures that open the lungs and expand the upper back, beginning, for example, with a modified Shoulderstand (*Viparita Karani*), supported with bolsters.[6] She would also work with poses that stretch the student's intestines, like reclining Hero Pose (*Supta Virasana*).[7] A person whose spine is rounded forward might have difficulty with backbending poses. Karin will work slowly, supporting a student in restorative postures on the floor, using bolsters to lift the chest and open the lungs. After a number of sessions, she might introduce backbends by doing the work herself, lifting her client's upper body into Cobra (*Bhujangasana*).

Karin, like most Iyengar teachers, might *not* begin with teaching Robert pranayama breathing exercises, as would teachers from some other traditions. "Iyengar's approach," she says, "has always been that you prepare the lungs to receive the breath." This means staying in a restorative pose like Smiling Heart Pose, described in the Yoga Experience at the end of Chapter Two. Iyengar's philosophy, "preparing the lungs to receive the breath," follows the Classical Yoga approach to the Eight-Limbed Path—climbing from one limb to another, like rungs of a ladder, up the Yoga tree.

I agree with Karin that starting in a restorative pose like Smiling Heart is a good way to invigorate the lungs with blood flow and increased oxygen. If your solar plexus is tight and your lungs are constricted, beginning your practice in a restorative pose can help introduce more breath into the lungs. My approach to working with the breath is a little different from Karin's and those of most Iyengar teachers. In the tradition of Yoga I practice and teach, we do not wait so long to introduce the breath. Whether you are depressed or anxious, I believe that you will benefit from working with the breath, using pranayama breathing exercises even as you are just beginning a practice of postures. In fact, as we'll learn in Chapter Seven, hospitalized patients in India had a significant recovery rate from major depression when they learned only one breathing exercise, *Sudharshan Kriya*, with no postures or meditation. However, as was the case with Janis Carter's patients who suffered from PTSD, many Iyengar students have seen their symptoms improve without working directly with the breath.

Karin Stephan works individually with students who suffer from depression, designing a practice that is both grounded in her intuition—that "angled light" reading of a client's needs—and her many years of practicing and teaching Iyengar Yoga. Her colleague, senior Iyengar teacher Patricia Walden, also specializes in working with people suffering from depression, leading national workshops on Yoga for depression that basically follow B.K.S. Iyengar's prescription of postures, though Patricia adds some simple breathing exercises.

In general, for people suffering from dysthymia, which Patricia characterizes as inertia or a sense of hopelessness (tamasic), Patricia recommends a vigorous Iyengar practice. She works with this group of students in an active way, presenting them with a physically challenging sequence of postures that keeps them "out of themselves." Like Karin's plan for Robert's recovery, Patricia recommends backbends and inversions. She tells her depressed students to keep their eyes open wide and to keep moving from posture to posture without pausing in between. "When a student is depressed," she says, "you don't want him brooding. You want him to keep moving, generating life force in his body. You want her to feel breath moving through her body, making her feel alive." Patricia also recommends supported backbends that open the chest and get the adrenal glands pumping. For people suffering from this kind of depression, Patricia doesn't encourage seated forward bends. "If you're already feeling empty and lethargic, sitting with the head down, so still and quiet, can make you feel worse." After a strong practice, she recommends a brief cool-down. Instead of relaxing in Corpse Pose (Shavasana), if someone is severely depressed, she recommends Reclining Bound Angle Pose (*Supta Baddhakonasana*),[8] a cooling-down posture done with the back, neck, and head supported, the eyes open, and the knees separated and propped on a bolster.

Students whose depression is combined with anxiety often have trouble being still and quieting down. They, too, benefit from a hard workout followed by a long cool-down. She suggests Bridge Pose (*Setu Bandhasana*)[9] toward the end of practice as well as forward bends, followed by a long relaxation in Corpse Pose (Shavasana). Though a student with an anxiety depression would have a hard time settling into Corpse Pose at the beginning of practice, after an energetic workout a long relaxation in Corpse Pose feels wonderful.

Patricia agrees with Yoga teachers and therapists from other traditions that a person suffering from depression will do better practicing in a class than trying to maintain a practice without the support of the group and an inspiring teacher. "The kind of yoga you practice is secondary to the kind of teacher you find," says Patricia. "It's important to find a teacher who uses language to inspire, building self-esteem in direct and indirect ways."

Viniyoga—Meeting It All

In Chapter One, we talked about meeting the depression—how important it is to ascertain your mood and meet it; to stay attuned to the breath and movement, slowly easing yourself in the opposite direction, bringing balance to the emotional and physical body. When you are observing your mood, in order to determine the direction of your practice, you are already engaged in self-study (svadhyaya), essential to the Viniyoga approach to treating depression, which works with the qualities of your nature (the gunas), discussed earlier, to bring balance back into your system.

You know that when you are flattened out by your depression, Yoga, particularly an active practice, may be the last thing you feel capable of, even if it might be the best thing you could do for yourself. On the other hand, if you're feeling anxious, your active, jumpy mind may not be able to tolerate a deep, slow practice, though such a soothing experience might benefit you. A Viniyoga teacher will work with you individually to design a practice that addresses all the places you need to bring into balance, physically, mentally, and emotionally. A Viniyoga approach enters through the doorway of self-observation (svadhyaya) to find the balance of willful practice (tapas) and surrender (Ishvara-pranidhana).

Viniyoga is a tradition of Yoga in the lineage of the great Yoga master Krishnamacharya, whose son, T.K.V. Desikachar, continues that tradition. Many Yoga therapists in the West practice and teach within this tradition, which adapts Yoga practice to the needs of the individual. "In Viniyoga, we work with the whole person, not the symptom," says Gary Kraftsow, director of American Viniyoga and author of two excellent books about Viniyoga, *Yoga for Wellness: Healing with the Timeless Teachings of Viniyoga* and *Yoga for Transformation: Ancient Teachings and Practices for Healing the Body, Mind and Heart*. "We don't see a depressed person but a person who has depression."

The therapeutic treatment in Viniyoga is based on the two governing concepts of Ayurveda medicine, the first of which is *langhana*. Langhana techniques in Yoga reduce, eliminate, calm, and purify. Typically, when practicing a posture to calm the system, it might be held a little longer, as you continue to breathe. These techniques are appropriate for someone suffering from an anxiety-based depression (rajasic). On the other hand, *brahmana* techniques in Yoga nourish, build, and energize. Typically, an energizing practice for someone suffering from dysthymia (tamasic) might use repetitive movements. You may, for example, move in and out of the posture several times, using the breath rather than holding it in a steady position. "It is important to remember," Gary says, "that each individual is unique, and that all techniques should be adapted to the needs of the individual body's structure. Viniyoga's view is that it is the job of the teacher to provide the appropriate method for the student and not be fixated on one modality."[10]

Treatment of depression in the Viniyoga may go beyond the bounds of ordinary Hatha Yoga practice. Gary will often suggest that a person with depression take on charitable work and spend time playing with children. "Something wonderful happens to you when you make a child happy," he says. For a woman with depression who lives in Los Angeles, Gary suggested that she first take an early-morning walk on the beach, then do her yoga practice, followed by a healthy breakfast. He also suggested that she join the Sierra Club and go on hikes with others. He recognized that her whole way of living had to shift, that she needed to reconnect with nature and with friends, and that wouldn't happen through asana practice alone. "The first step for many people is not a link with God, as much as the link with *satsanga,* with others in a spiritual community, who view life positively."

The basis for making these adjustments in a person's activities is not to add something that is missing in a person's system, but to break through the obstacles to the person's experience of themselves. In the Viniyoga approach, transformation occurs not by adding or taking away, but by adjusting and balancing the basic qualities of our nature.

"When I'm working with breathing or with the body," says Leslie Kaminoff, a Yoga therapist who uses Viniyoga techniques in his work with clients, "my confidence is that the system has its own power to seek equilibrium and to heal. I don't have to put into the system anything that's missing. I just have to help the person find what's obstructing them. It's similar to what a farmer does when he breaks a dam to let water flow to his crops." The principle, then, is one of simply removing obstructions, to free up the space.

Kripalu Yoga—Embracing It All

From its inception, Kripalu Yoga has been a practice that combines will-ful practice (tapas) with self-study (svadhyaya) and the cultivation of sur-render (Ishvara-pranidhana) in a system of meditation-in-motion developed in the early 1970s by Yogi Amrit Desai.

Swami Kripalvanandji, who was Desai's teacher and is considered to be the "grandfather" of Kripalu Yoga, understood that self-study (svadh-yaya) is not only as important as willful practice, but is an essential aspect of Yoga. "Self-observation without judgment is the highest spiritual prac-tice," he often said. He also understood the importance of surrender. His own story is one of surrender, first, to the depths of darkest depression, then to a path out of the darkness and into the light. Swami Kripal-vanandji, known also as Swami Kripalu and to his disciples as Bapuji, was so despondent in his early twenties that he nearly ended his life. At the brink of suicide, a divine Yogic intervention in the form of a sanyasin (renunciate, or one who has renounced the pleasures of the senses), who Swami Kripalu came to believe was a divine manifestation of the ancient Lord Lakulish, saved and transformed his life. He surrendered himself to learning all that he could from this mysterious Yogi. The *Pashupat* lineage he embraced is a *Tantric* path that traces its roots to the actual historical figure of Lord Lakulish, a contemporary of Patanjali's, who was probably one of the earliest teachers to refine the practices of Yoga.

Tantric philosophy is essentially nondualist. The belief is that the Absolute is everywhere, that our feelings of separation are only an illu-sion. All the practices in Kripalu Yoga are simply tools to strip away the layers of armoring that keep us feeling separate from ourselves and oth-ers. This philosophy is the basis for looking to Yoga as a way to heal the heart. "You are born divine," said Swami Kripalu and his disciple Yogi Amrit Desai. It is only our ignorance (avidya) that keeps us believing we are separate.

The actual practice of Kripalu Yoga moves the practitioner from willful holding, through self-observation, into a total surrender to spon-taneous movements while releasing the pose. In his many hours of daily practice, Swami Kripalu often went into ecstatic states of spontaneous postures and *mudras* (hand gestures that seal cosmic energy within the mind, body, and heart of the practitioner). And Kripalu Yoga as a formal practice was born when, in early-morning Yoga practice (*sadhana*) with his wife and friends, Amrit Desai began moving spontaneously, surrendering to the energy his posture and pranayama session had generated. Senior Kripalu teachers refined the process of moving from willful practice through self-observation to surrender in their development of the three stages of Kripalu Yoga practiced today.

A Kripalu Yoga class is a creative session that can be taught gently, moderately, or vigorously. At every level, there is an emphasis on the breath and on listening to the sensations in your body. You can expect to learn pranayama, asana, and a short form of centering meditation in a Kripalu Yoga class. There is no prescribed sequence of postures in a Kripalu class, as one might find in an Ashtanga or Bikram class. Paying attention to the ability level of the students and the energy in the room, a Kripalu teacher creates a sequence of poses for each class that moves and stretches the body in all directions and includes forward bending, backbending, side stretching, twists, and usually, though not always in a beginning class, an inversion.

Each of the three stages of Kripalu Yoga aligns with and strengthens one leg of the Yoga tripod. Whether the class you take is gentle or vigorous, a Kripalu-trained teacher may offer an experience of all three stages of the practice. In Stage I the emphasis is on the willful practice of a pose (tapas), focusing on details of alignment. In Stage II, the focus is on self-study (svadhyaya) as you observe the sensations in your body, your feelings, and your thoughts in a longer-than-usual holding of a pose. In Stage III, the focus is on Ishvara-pranidhana as you completely surrender to the flow of energy in your body while spontaneously releasing from the held pose. Throughout the release and for several minutes afterward, you may be guided to follow the sensations of your body into a flow of movements.

In every stage, the emphasis is on developing a sense of "Witness Consciousness," watching, with ever-growing self-awareness and equanimity, the sensations in the physical body and the thoughts and feelings that rise in the mind. As Witness Consciousness grows, you begin to accept yourself as you are and make peace with reality as it is.

It was this self-accepting attitude that I encountered when I first walked through the doors of Kripalu Center in 1989. And it is this self-accepting attitude that has kept me practicing through personal loss, my bout with breast cancer, and mistakes I have made along the way. It is that self-accepting attitude that I believe was the foundation of my recovery from depression, and it is what strengthens my capacity to move through adversity. Every time I step onto my Yoga mat, it is a gesture of self-acceptance, a gesture of loving myself just as I am, with whatever stiffness or discomfort I show up with that day. Every time I step onto my mat, I am honoring my body, just as it is, as though it were a temple of the divine. And it is. Because when I practice and the tensions in my body begin to melt away and the clinging thoughts begin to dissolve, I am left with the knowledge of who I really am. I am aware of my own divinity and the divinity of all beings, and in this awareness, I no longer feel separate and alone.

But how did I get from a person suffering from depression, a person whose therapist told her she would always be "one of those people with empty pockets," to feeling so abundant, so grateful to be alive, to be a part of the reality that is here and now? The truth is, *I don't know!* I know the research and medical evidence about what Yoga does—it's all there in Chapter Three. I know what Yogis whose knowledge I respect say—their wisdom is scattered throughout this book. I know a little of what the ancient Yoga texts say—I've studied the *Yoga Sutras*, the *Bhagavad Gita*, and the *Hatha Yoga Pradipika*. All of them point to one thing—Yoga as the science of positive mental health will bring whatever is out of balance in your physical, your emotional, and your mental body back into balance. But *how, exactly, did it happen to me?*

I grew up believing the image I carried of myself inside was, despite my appearance, who I *really* was. And inside, for most of my life, I have been a dark, chubby little Jewish girl from the Northeast. This image was real to me, despite the reality that I have always been fair and, though I have had cycles of compulsive overeating, I have never been seriously overweight. After practicing Yoga for several years, I was given a Sanskrit name. The name chosen for me by Amrit Desai was "Divyajyoti," a big, wonderful name that means "Divine Light." For a time at Kripalu and in India, I was known to my friends as Divyajyoti. There is even an auto rickshaw driven by my Indian friends through the streets of Ooty in the state of Tamil Nadu, with my name painted on the back! But how could I, a dark, chubby little Jewish girl from the Northeast, live up to such a name? I loved it, of course. Answering to a short little (chubby?) name like Amy all my life, I felt longer and more graceful as I walked through the world bearing such an elegant and important name. I told myself that though I certainly didn't deserve it, Divyajyoti was a name to grow into. And over time, practicing Yoga every day, I think I did.

For a number of years, I was in a relationship with a man who was a white, Anglo-Saxon Protestant from the Midwest. He was tall and handsome and had light hair and blue eyes. Inside, I asked myself what I, the dark, chubby little Jewish girl from the Northeast, could be doing with such a person. What a surprise it was to me when the new friends we met when we moved to Tucson so often commented on how much we looked alike! Had I grown into my name? Yes, I think I actually had. I no longer go by Divyajyoti, but over the years of my practice, I have filled up with my name. When I step onto my mat I am "Divine Light," and more and more, I carry that light with me wherever I go. A dark, chubby little Jewish girl still lives inside me, and she is surrounded by Divine Light.

I've written my way back to the question: *How did it happen? How did I become a happy person?* I still don't know, but if I talk about what my experience is like on my mat, you will see how I move through all three stages of practice, and perhaps we'll both understand my recovery.

My Yoga Practice

This is an experience of my Yoga session now, not what it was like when I started. Back then, I followed a teacher's lead, either in class or from an audiotape. Almost always, I felt both relaxed and energized after my practice. Sometimes, even in my first few months of practice, I felt moments of bliss in a posture or its release, little glimpses of my own authentic nature, my wholeness. At times there were tears, often for no reason—simply energy releasing in my body. I moved off my mat, often inspired, ready to begin my day.

Fifteen years after I began a daily practice, I come to my mat each morning from the stiffness of sleep, with dream images floating in my mind. Sometimes, in the background, I play inspiring music, but more often I prefer silence or the natural sounds of my neighborhood waking outside my window. I usually begin in Child Pose, with my hips on my heels, my forehead on the mat, and my arms extended over my head, my hands in prayer. In a way, I am actually beginning in a posture of surrender, cultivating the vulnerability, the curiosity, the enthusiasm, and the receptivity of a child. I may stay here for just a moment or for several minutes, setting an intention for my practice or asking for something that I feel I need. Usually, these days, I ask to simply be allowed to always feel the presence of the divine—in my breath, in the sensations in my body, in my thoughts and feelings. I ask to remember that God is with me, even in the stiffness in my hip, the queasy feeling in my belly—yes, that is God telling me I shouldn't have eaten that sugary Congo bar last night!—or my somber mood. Sometimes I ask for clarity or help in holding to some personal resolve. Sometimes I will use an affirmation, like the one I suggested in Chapter Two: "Thou art with me. Thank you." Often I think of something I am especially grateful for that day, and always I express my gratitude for my body, which is still healthy and strong enough to practice Yoga every day. In a kind of prayer, I offer my thanks for the practice and for all the teachers who have influenced my life, beginning with my first guru, Louise, my next-door neighbor when I was growing up, who taught me that love is what matters most.

By now I know whether I need to begin standing or if I need a slower entry into my practice. It's no longer a conscious thought like "I have a lot of energy this morning, so I want to start with Sun Salutations." My body just begins with the practices it is drawn to, and I follow along. Most often, in the morning, I do not start standing, as I might in the afternoon. From Child Pose, I find my way onto my hands and knees in table position, to practice the Six Movements of the Spine as I described them in the Yoga Experience in Chapter Two. As I move, I do so with deep breaths in and out through my nostrils. I take time to undulate my spine, to circle my hips, noticing areas of tightness, areas where energy may be blocked in my body. I consciously breathe into those areas of tension, inviting them to relax.

After warming up my spine, I may do some leg stretches, sometimes from table position, sometimes lying on my back, sometimes from sitting. I may tighten and release the muscles in my shoulders and back, and I may rotate my head and stretch my neck. If I notice any other areas of tension in my body, I might do a warm-up stretch to release the tightness there. Lately, I've been working on the tendons in my calves. I ride a bike, and I've noticed an increasing tightness there. So I may sit for some time in a squatting position, with my feet close together, my heels reaching for the floor. I might also sit in a chair and, with my feet pigeon-toed, lean forward toward my feet.

Eventually, I come through a few moments in Rag Doll, with my knees slightly bent, letting the tension roll off my spine, into a standing position. Here, I may do some vigorous breathing exercises, like the "Power Hara," or "Breath of Joy," or "Uddiyana Bandha and Agni Sara," described in the Yoga Experience in Chapter Six. After the vigorous breathing, I close my eyes to feel the effects, noticing where my energy is flowing freely, noticing where it may still be blocked. I may practice another breathing exercise with special attention to the area of tightness, then pause to notice my energy again. Usually, by this point in my practice, I feel my energy expanding beyond the boundaries of my physical body. And I think to myself how much bigger I am than this body, this mind, these emotions. I feel my wholeness in these moments and remember my intention for my practice. Then I ground this expanded energy in my standing practice.

I plant my feet directly beneath me and parallel, my big toes touching, and stand with my spine erect, my shoulder blades drawn down my back, and my crown lifted. I let my palms face out, so that I can feel the energy running through me—the energy I am sending out into the universe and the energy I am receiving. Then I lift my arms slowly, observing the sensations in my body. I come into Mountain Pose, as I describe it in the Yoga Experience in Chapter Three. I stand for several moments, feeling my alignment, my energy. Am I grounded? Is my energy aligned with the energy of the universe? Do I feel supported by this energy? I might ask again for clarity and support in my intention for that day. I will take several long deep breaths, expanding my lungs with life breath. Then I draw my hands together slowly over my head, feeling the energy between my palms. Sometimes I let my fingertips touch, circling them for a moment, giving myself the gift of that sweet sensation before I interlace my fingers with my index fingers extended. I will frame my ears with my straight arms and practice a deep stretch to the right and left, holding for several breaths on each side, noticing the tightness or ease in my hips and my shoulders. Sometimes, if my lower back feels ready, I will practice an easy backbend, paying attention to engaging my leg muscles, keeping the muscles firm in my thoracic spine, drawing my lower abdomen in toward my spine in order to protect my lower back, and lifting up and out of my chest. But sometimes it feels too early in my practice for a backbend, so I forgo it and practice a strong forward bend with a flat back. Here I might hold my ankles or slip my hands under my heels or under my toes, giving myself a stretch along the whole back side of my body. From here I might step my right leg back into Runner's Stretch, with my left knee directly over my ankle. From this position I will practice a series of leg stretches. Then I will step my left leg back to meet my right and hold myself up in a plank position, sometimes bending my elbows and lowering toward the floor for more of a challenge. In this position I will practice an energizing breath like Skull Shining (*Kapalabhati*), described in the Yoga Experience in Chapter Six.

From here I will continue to stretch, moving through many standing postures, balancing the energy by practicing the same sequence on both the right and left sides. I won't describe the specific postures, so as not to confuse you with poses you may not know. The routine includes several Warriors, Triangles, Side Angle Poses, Standing Twists, Squats, and balancing poses, all designed to strengthen and tone my body. Always when I practice, I am using the Ocean-Sounding Victory Breath (*Ujjayi*). I listen to my breath and it becomes like a lullaby to myself— the sound, like a wave over pebbles, soothes me, even as my body begins to tremble in a long holding of a Warrior Pose. Sometimes when I hold a posture like Warrior or Triangle, I may take support from a more vigorous breath like Skull Shining (Kapalabhati). Often when I'm holding, I may chant a mantra, or use an affirmation like "I stand firm in the energy of the universe, and the energy of the universe supports me." After perhaps twenty to thirty minutes of standing poses, I will come down, often releasing out of a standing posture into a flow of spontaneous movements, some of which may look like Yoga, some of which may look more like dance. I simply let my body and my awakened energy guide me into a flow of movements, eventually ending my flow on my back or my belly. There I rest for several minutes, balancing the vigorous part of my practice with quiet attention to all that's true in my physical body and my emotional body.

After my rest, I will practice backbends, twists, forward bends, and inversions for another twenty to thirty minutes, often varying the sequence and my choice of poses. I practice each pose with Ocean-Sounding Breath, listening to the sensations in my body, tracing the feelings that rise and fall, without judgment about any of it. I am cultivating both equanimity and awareness as I practice, developing a capacity to accept my body exactly the way it is showing up on the mat on this day. This is the Witness Consciousness that grows with the practice of Yoga. With this Witness comes a growing sense of serenity, an acceptance of reality, not as I wish it to be but exactly as it is. This is a source of my ever-expanding happiness.

Eventually I may hold a pose that is challenging for me. I might choose to hold it beyond the point where my body begins to tremble and feel the discomfort of the position. It is here that I can see where in my body I need to open more, what I need to release more, and perhaps I'll have an awareness of where in my life off the mat I may need to hold on and where I may need to let go. I breathe into the strong sensations, I consciously relax the areas of tension, I feel all that is present in my physical body and my emotional body, and I allow myself to accept all of it. As I release, I notice how the areas of tension in my body become areas of pleasure, how my body floods with sensation and energy, with my awareness of the divine. Again I move into a spontaneous flow of movement, a dance of Yoga, letting the divinity within guide me, until I trust my body to bring me down on my back in Corpse Pose. I may tuck a cushion under my knees, place an eye bag over my eyes, and perhaps pull a blanket up around me. I may stay in Corpse Pose for about ten minutes, sometimes merely resting, sometimes in a healing state, where I am aware and alert but also deeply connected to all that is, a state where I am not a separate being but a part of the whole of the universe.

Sometimes in the middle of holding a pose I will have glimpses of this state. This is the deep, relaxing state in which the mind and body heal. This is a felt sense of my own divinity. Better than any SSRI, better than any drug, better even than chocolate or sex. This is why I practice.

For many years, this was the end of my practice. This, in a shorter, more moderate, beginner's version, was all I did to recover from depression. Now, however, I am continuing to practice for another thirty to forty minutes, not to heal from depression but to maintain and expand my awareness of the truth of my existence, my wholeness, throughout my day. These extra minutes provide ever-increasing access to that healing state, those glimpses into reality that the Yogis call samadhi. In this part of my session, I practice about twenty minutes of pranayama breathing exercises, after which I may meditate for up to twenty minutes. Most often, when my meditation is complete, I burst into spontaneous song, sometimes simply sounding tones, sometimes singing my favorite mantra: *Om namo bhagavate Vasudevaya*—Thy will, O Lord, not mine.

So how did I move from being "one of those people with empty pockets" to feeling abundant and full of gratitude almost all of the time? It wasn't the length or depth of my practice; nor was it the vigorous breathing techniques and the advanced postures. Truthfully, I began feeling better when I was new to Yoga, a beginner learning basic postures and simple breathing exercises, and yes, learning to listen and to accept my body, practicing for less than an hour *every day*. Do you see? Can you recognize the words in that sentence that made the biggest difference in my life? Those words are "every day." It was the intention to attend to myself, to accept myself just as I showed up on my mat *every day*, that allowed me to begin to embrace it all—the dark, chubby little Jewish girl from the Northeast, the "Divine Light," the "empty pockets," and the abundance—to embrace all of it with love.

yoga experience

The posture in this Yoga Experience is more advanced than what I have offered so far; however, it can be modified for beginners. I include Camel Pose here because it is so beneficial for depression. After practicing this posture, you will feel lighter, brighter, and ready for what life brings.

Camel Pose (Ustrasansa)

Camel Pose opens and expands the chest, lifts the spirits, and increases lung capacity and blood circulation throughout the body. Try this posture only after you have warmed the body with gentle stretching for the muscles and flexing for the joints. You may wish to practice several exercises on your hands and knees. The Six Movements for the Spine, described in the Yoga Experience section at the end of Chapter Two, are good warm-ups to prepare the body for Camel Pose. However, Camel Pose is best practiced toward the end of your posture sequence, after the body is thoroughly stretched and relaxed.

Come into a kneeling position. Before you begin, roll your shoulders up and back several times, then reverse the direction, using the breath (inhaling up, exhaling down). This helps release the tension in your shoulders. Place your hands on your hips and slowly rotate your hips in one direction and then the other, noticing any tight places in your lower back. If there is tightness or soreness there, do not practice this pose, or modify it as I describe below.

Place your palms on your sacrum with your fingers pointed down. Lift your chest and, if it is comfortable, let your head drop back. Press your pelvis forward and arch your back. This is the modified pose, and you may hold right here, continuing to breathe long and deep through the nostrils.

If you wish to move into the full pose, lean back and place your right hand on your right heel, your left hand on your left heel. Keep pressing your pelvis forward and lifting your chest so that the weight of your body is not in your hands. Lifting the chest or sternum elongates the lumbar spine and reduces the curve, making the posture safer and reducing the feeling of compression there. Breathe long and deep through the nostrils. Hold for twenty seconds, coming out earlier if the sensation grows too strong, staying a little longer if your body wishes a deeper experience. *Listen to your body.* (As an alternative, you might give yourself a comfortable backbend by draping your back over a large exercise ball with your feet planted firmly on the floor. Or place the ball against the wall and with your feet planted on the floor, lean back, reaching for the wall with your hands.) This is a posture that stimulates the thymus gland, and it is an excellent immune system builder. Camel Pose expands the chest and opens the heart.

To come out of the pose, slowly move your right hand to your lower back, then your left hand. When you feel complete, rest in Child Pose with your hips on your heels and your forehead on the floor. After stretching your arms in front of you for an extension of your spine, let your arms come alongside your body to relax your shoulders. You may wish to gently rock across your forehead, stimulating the pituitary gland behind your third eye.

When you are ready, return to a sitting position, close your eyes, and notice how you feel.

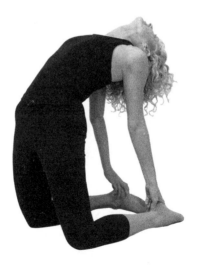

Camel Pose (Ustrasansa)

CHAPTER SIX

fire in the belly—managing with yogic breathing

In the breath, the soul
finds an opportunity to speak.

—DANNA FAULDS, from "Breath"[1]

In 1999, cancer cells were removed from my right breast in a core
biopsy. I was fortunate: The surgery that followed did not reveal
more cancer, so my recovery did not involve either chemotherapy or
radiation. Still, in the weeks between the core biopsy and the surgery, I
felt a multitude of emotions—fear, disbelief, panic, grief. I let these feelings surface, particularly on my Yoga mat, where my practice would
bring balance back into my emotional body. My pranayama practice
was especially valuable during this time. I had a direct experience of

working with my breath, managing my *prana* to manage my feelings. I will explain how I did this, but first let's look at the concept of Prana.

Prana

In many ways, the cosmic energy that is Prana corresponds to that of modern nuclear physics, "which regards all matter as energy 'organized' in different ways."[2] This is Prana with a capital *P*. It is the Prana that knows no boundaries. Its source is the energy of the universe, that which is unchanging within you, your very soul, and it feeds your energy body, what the ancient texts call the *pranamayakosha*. Prana (small *p*) refers to the energy in the atmosphere—oxygen-rich air. This prana, also known as *vayu*, feeds the physical body, what the ancient Yogis call the *annamayakosha*.

The ancient Yogis on the trail of enlightenment didn't think in terms of oxygen-rich air. These holy ones (*sadhus*) were more likely to withdraw from the world of externals, including beauty and health, and, says senior Kripalu teacher Yoganand Michael Carroll, "might as easily practice in a cremation ground, a cave, or a small hut with walls smeared with cow dung." However, modern Yogis are more health conscious and more often live lives not of withdrawal but of community. We are more interested in positive mental health than in liberation. And so we take ourselves out to nature to be inspired and to breathe the prana-rich air. Like most modern practitioners, I believe that there are varying amounts of prana available in different climates and geographical locations. You may feel invigorated by prana in more turbulent zones—high mountains, for instance, or by the sea. Think about where, on vacation or in your daily life, you have felt most revitalized. For me, my barefoot walks along the beaches of Rhode Island, my dawn Yoga practice while camping on a mountain in Sedona, my afternoon walks, often barefoot, along the paths of the Nilgiris Mountains in Tamil Nadu, were times when my spirit was refreshed and the manifestation of my prana seemed most aligned with the cosmic Prana of the universe.

Obviously, there is less prana available in the artificial atmosphere of an office building than in the broad sweep of the desert. If you are someone who lives in a high-rise, commutes underground, and works in an office building, your depression may be magnified by the reduction in atmospheric prana. How often do your feet actually touch the earth? Think about it. Go to the rooftop on your lunch break, walk home in the sun if you can, crossing through a park where your feet can briefly have access to the earth, and take vacations to prana-rich environments like the seaside or the mountains.

For most of us who use computers and cell phones and watch television, the environment in which we work and play can contribute not only to a disturbance in our bioenergetic field, but to a kind of prana starvation. We often don't realize the extent to which our systems are deprived of prana. Senior Yoga teacher and founder of the American Yoga College Rama Jyoti Vernon believes that modern life—what we do, what we eat, what we breathe—is contributing to a rise in depression and hopelessness, particularly among young people. Not only the air we breathe, but also much of the water we drink and the food we eat, is deprived of the nutrients we need to feel healthy and filled with prana. "The soil has become so depleted," says Rama, "that we're losing the vitamins and minerals that can contribute to a balanced chemistry of the body and the mind." We may not be able to move to the mountains, but we can use Yogic methods to enrich our prana, wherever we live.

Naturally High

When we look around us, it seems that some people have more prana than others. They naturally seem to exude energy. We gravitate to such people. My friend Dena Baumgartner, a renowned psychodramatist, is such a being. Wherever she goes—a market in New Orleans, a workshop in Latvia, a restaurant in Tucson—people are drawn to her energy. She has no regular spiritual practice and pranayama breathing exercises are not easy for her. Yet she exudes prana and is a source of energizing prana for others. If our own prana is a personal reservoir for universal prana, it is difficult to understand why some of us have more innate prana, or *qi,* as the Chinese call our life force, than others. According to Yoga scholar Kurt Keutzer, some Chinese texts distinguish between "innate qi," the energy we have at birth, and "cultivated qi," the energy that can be developed. Clearly, some people simply have more "innate" prana. This manifests as "a stronger more resilient body and greater general vitality."[3] All Eastern traditions believe that our energy reservoir can be strengthened. When we clear away the obstacles to the free flow of thought and feeling through regular Yoga and pranayama breathing practice, we can revitalize our prana.

Mood Management with Pranayama

Prana in the form of breath is our vital energy, our life force. In many ancient cultures, the word or phrase that means breath also means spirit or soul. In Hebrew that word is *ruach*; in Greek, *psyche pneuma*; in Japanese, *ki*. When we restrict the breath, we are diminishing the spirit. When we relearn to breathe fully and deeply, we are enlarging the spirit and reconnecting with the Self. When we are breathing consciously, we remember who we are.

Prana is to the body what gasoline is to a car, electricity to a light-bulb, wind to a windmill. *Pranayama* means the "control of life breath." Learning pranayama breathing exercises is like learning to drive a car—when to accelerate, when to brake. The ancient Yogis understood that when you can consciously regulate the breath, you can manage your feelings and moods by accelerating your energy or by putting on the brakes. Harnessing prana through pranayama breathing exercises gives you tremendous power at your solar plexus. It's like revving up your engine, moving from six horsepower to sixty. When we consciously control the breath, we are directing, through the power of our thought, the current of prana.

During the time I faced cancer, I had direct experience of my own ability to manage my feelings with my breath. In the beginning, when I first heard the news, I needed to decelerate. I practiced two calming pranayama breathing exercises that you will find in the Yoga Experience at the end of this chapter. Ocean-Sounding Victory Breath (Ujjayi) was my staple through the day as well as Alternate-Nostril Breathing (Nadi Sodhana). The long, deep breaths I took calmed the fear, and the slow Alternate-Nostril Breaths eased the anxious feelings I was experiencing.

During the surgery, I was placed under a general anesthetic. Afterward, I felt listless and weak for days. After several weeks, the lethargy and low mood began to feel like depression. I needed to accelerate my energy. I decided to experiment in my practice, introducing more and longer periods of energizing breaths like Skull-Shining Breath (Kapalab-hati), described in the Yoga Experience.

I also began to more consciously practice compassion toward myself, accepting even this dull and sluggish self. When I was told I had cancer, my mind worked overtime, trying to make sense of the diagnosis. Was it my diet? Was it old, unprocessed emotions I had transcended prema-turely in my spiritual quest? Was it the high dose of estrogen I took daily when I was a teenager, in order to regulate my period? I knew, of course, that such questions are irrelevant to life in the twenty-first century, when one American woman in eight will get breast cancer. Still, the questions persisted. If only I had stopped eating meat sooner. If only I'd washed my nonorganic produce more thoroughly. If only I'd gone organic years ago. If only I'd done another Inner Quest Intensive,[4] given myself permission to feel angry, done a ten-day sit every year, dealt more consciously with my sexuality. Not for the first time in my life I remem-bered Swami Kripalu's words, words I heard repeated in my first pro-gram at Kripalu Center—*My beloved child, break your heart no longer. Each time you judge yourself, you break your own heart.* Then I could stop, take a deep Ocean-Sounding Victory Breath, and release into an acceptance of the clouded sky of my energy. This will pass, I told myself. Blue sky exists beneath the weather of my current mood.

As I worked with my breath—experimenting with pranayama—and my thoughts—using affirmations and cognitive therapy exercises from *The Feeling Good Handbook Workbook* by David Burns, M.D., to counter-act my negative thinking—I was able to accept the scared little girl inside, the suddenly sluggish middle-aged woman, and my body that would not always be trim and fit and healthy, my body that is continuing to change as I grow older.

The Breath as Metaphor

In my experience with cancer, I was able to regulate my mood by work-ing consciously with the breath. Most of the time, we are breathing unconsciously, automatically, and not necessarily in a way that is serving our good feelings about ourselves. Let's look at the way we automatically breathe and why managing the breath can make such a difference. When we were born, we breathed with our entire bodies. Each breath was like a wave that brought a wake of movement along the spine, down to the tailbone. But as we grew older, fear, sadness, anger, and other emotional states changed the way we breathed. We began to restrict the breath in response to the darker emotions, and little by little we forgot the most natural way to breathe. Our respiratory system continued to function mechanically, drawing in oxygen and releasing carbon dioxide from the constricted arena of our lungs. But as our capacity to breathe fully diminished, so did our ability to experience the enthusiasms and joys of childhood.

The way in which you breathe is a metaphor for the way in which you are living your life. Are you taking little sips of breath as though you don't have permission to take up much space on the planet? One of my Yoga students told me that for years she, unbeknownst even to herself, lived only to please others. Joan told me that she wasn't a character, even in her most private moments—her own sexual fantasies. In lovemaking, she often felt numb or rode on her husband's passion, which she believes was triggered by pornography, not by his passion for her. Joan was the woman at the party whose name you cannot remember. Even if she arrived early for Yoga class, she set her mat up in the back of the room. Joan's breath was nearly imperceptible. When students are folded into Child Pose (hips on the heels, forehead resting on the mat), I sometimes give back presses, watching and coordinating my touch with the movement of breath along a student's spine. Joan's respiration was so shallow, I could not easily find it.

It was not easy for Joan to learn to breathe deeply and slowly into her lungs. But over time, with practice, her breathing improved. Later, after she had been practicing pranayama breathing exercises for nearly a year, she told me how angry she was feeling about the way she had been living, how over and over, for as long as she could remember, she'd played such a bit part in her life that her name wasn't even on the marquee. Though it was her fifty-year-old body that climbed out of bed in the morning, her husband and her children directed and starred in her life. As Joan began to control her breath through her pranayama practice, she began to take control of her life. "When he gets aroused from looking at a sexy magazine, I can say 'no' to him now," she told me, describing her husband's ardor. "On the other hand, I can sense when it's about me, about us, and I can respond with more passion."

Although Joan had always considered herself a feminist and had been in consciousness-raising groups in the seventies, women's ritual groups in the eighties, and a book group in the nineties, she always took a backseat in the group's organization and activities and rarely hosted a meeting. After a year of pranayama practice, Joan founded her own women's group, and though the format was similar to others—an hour or so of individual sharing, followed by an experience or ritual initiated by one of the members—Joan always led a breathing exercise to begin the group. "When I lead a pranayama like Alternate-Nostril Breathing, I am more grounded in my body, more connected to my feelings, and can really listen to me for a change. Then, when I check in, I can talk about myself rather than my husband or my children."

Leo, a high-rolling day trader who had been heavily invested in technology stocks, came to his first Yoga class several days after another downturn in the market. He was a natural athlete, but derived little pleasure from the competitive way he played. Often, in class, I could hear a deep sighing. His natural form of breathing seemed to be an unconscious retention followed by a mournful sigh. When I asked him about this after class, he confided that he hadn't been sleeping well, that his digestion was terrible, that he had irritable bowel syndrome (IBS), and that he was beset with personal problems he couldn't talk about. I suggested that he focus on Ocean-Sounding Victory Breath (Ujjayi), consciously listening to the sound, and trying to make the inhalations and exhalations smooth, with the exhalation slightly longer than the inhalation. I recommended that he practice breathing this way whenever he thought about it, both on and off the mat. I also suggested that he not practice Skull Shining Breath (Kapalabhati) or other breathing exercises that might stimulate too much energy in his lower chakras, which could further irritate his digestive tract. What he needed were calming, soothing breaths. After several weeks, he told me that though his problems were mounting, he was coping with them better. His sleep and his digestion were more regulated than before, and though he still had occasional flare-ups, even his IBS seemed better. "Now, if you could teach this breath to my wife and the guy who's suing me, we'd all be a lot happier," he said with a rueful laugh. Learning to control your breath won't solve all your problems, but it can help you cope with them better.

Breathing Basics

"I just realized that I really don't know how to breathe." I hear this often after students encounter their constricted breath during their first experience of Yoga. Even with clear instruction, it takes many weeks of practice before some students can actually breathe fully all the way to the bottom of their lungs, and even longer for some to be able to rapidly pump their bellies toward their spines in an energizing exercise like Skull-Shining Breath (Kapalabhati). What does knowing how to breathe look like? It is breathing that moves like a wave through your body, originating in the diaphragm rather than the thoracic region of the chest. It is full and deep and calm. To breathe in this way, the body must be relaxed. When we consciously tense the muscles and hold the breath, there is a relaxed feeling that accompanies the release. So the simplest way to relax is by contracting the muscles while holding the breath, then letting the muscles and breath release completely.

How We Breathe

The actual process of respiration takes place within the cells of the body. Not only are your nose, trachea (windpipe), and lungs involved, but the process of transporting oxygen from the air and modifying it so that it's available to your cells also involves your circulatory system and the muscles in your chest. Mechanically, there are three ways in which we draw oxygen into the lungs. We can extend the diaphragm down, which feels like a deep breath into the belly. This is diaphragmatic breathing, and it is the most efficient means of exposing the blood in the capillaries to air. It also circulates oxygenated blood to the lower, gravity-dependent parts of the lungs. This is the way a newborn breathes, and it is most suited for efficient breathing in our normal, daily activities. "When the diaphragm moves in the luxurious expansions that mark full breathing," says senior Yoga teacher Donna Farhi, "all [the] organs are massaged, rolled, churned, and bathed in new blood, fluids, and oxygen."[5]

Unfortunately, most of us have forgotten how to breathe this way. Instead, many of us use thoracic breathing for most of our activities. When we are breathing into the chest, we are using thoracic breathing. This breath expands the rib cage, using the intercostals, the muscles located between the ribs. Chest breathing is not as efficient as diaphragmatic breathing, because the lower portions of the lungs are not exposed to air. According to Alan Hymes, M.D., writing on the mechanics of breathing in *Science of Breath: A Practical Guide*, coauthored with Swami Rama and Rudolph Ballentine, M.D., "Chest breathing requires more work to accomplish the same blood/gas mixing than does slow, deep, diaphragmatic breathing."[6] Chest breathing uses more oxygen and is ultimately more work for the heart. Often people we might call Type-A personalities, like Leo, are prone to this kind of breathing and tend to develop anxiety-based depression.

According to Alexander Lowen, M.D., the founder of Bioenergetics, a system that works with the body and the breath to release repressed emotions, many people actually immobilize their diaphragms, unconsciously trying to control powerful feelings of fear or aggression or sexual response, pushing those feelings out of awareness. "The suppression of feeling creates a predisposition to depression," says Lowen, "since it prevents the individual from relying on feelings as a guide to behavior."[7] Bioenergetics works with the breath and the body in treating depression. "Therapeutically, it is easier and more effective to work with a patient from the physical or energetic side of the personality than from the psychic or interest side. Anyone who has lived with or treated a depressed person knows how difficult it is to activate him by arousing his interest."[8]

We generally use the third type of inhalation, clavicular breathing, to good effect when we are pumping a bicycle up a hill or otherwise exercising hard. However, if you are taking shallow breaths, using only the upper regions of your lungs throughout your daily activities, you may experience tension in your shoulders, upper back, and neck. You may also be prone to headaches and tension in your jaw. Many temporomandibular joint syndrome (TMJ) sufferers are shallow, upper-chest breathers. Until she became aware of her breathing in Yoga class, Joan was a clavicular breather.

Donna Farhi equates upper-chest breathing to a feeling of "being in your head" and out of touch with your emotions. She says that when we breathe into the lower regions of the lungs, we feel more grounded and stable. "As you focus your attention [and breathing action] in the lower body you become more in touch with your 'gut feelings.'"[9] This is the reason that when Joan began to breathe more deeply throughout the day, her anger began to surface. With that long-repressed anger came a desire to be a more active player in the drama of her life.

Balancing Right and Left

In 1994, while studying pranayama at Vivekananda Kendra Yoga Research Foundation in Bangalore, India, I met Shirley Telles, Ph.D., one of India's leading researchers in the field of Yoga. At the time of my visit, Shirley gave me a recently published study she had coauthored that clearly demonstrated the very different physiological effects of breathing through the left nostril as compared to the right. Since then, she and her colleagues at Vivekananda Kendra have continued to study the effects of many Yoga techniques, including postures, pranayama breathing exercises, meditation, and mantra chanting. Their studies are published in international medical journals and are among the most encouraging news we have about the effectiveness of using controlled, patterned breathing to treat the symptoms of depression.

Mental illness is a state of imbalance, so Alternate-Nostril Breathing or Purifying Breath (*Nadhi Sodhana*), described in the Yoga Experience, is a good way to provide balance for the right/left hemispheres of the brain and to increase oxygen to the cerebral tissues, which likely increases blood flow to the brain tissue. Telles's research at Vivekanandra Kendra shows that right-nostril breathing has a stimulating effect on the body and mind, while left-nostril breathing has a calming effect.[10] It makes sense, then, that if someone is suffering from a major depressive episode, her energy might be expanded with right-nostril dominance breathing, in which you inhale through the right nostril and exhale through the left. On the other hand, if you are feeling anxiety, a few extra rounds of left-nostril dominance breathing will help.

Kevin Durkin's experience of depression is a dramatic example of what can happen when one nostril, particularly the right nostril, the more stimulating side, is blocked. A forty-six-year-old Yoga teacher and body worker in Denver, Colorado, Kevin was physiologically prana-deprived for most of his life. As a teenager, he was hospitalized for a near-fatal sinusitis attack; he took years of allergy shots, had two operations for his deviated right septum, and had many in-office sinus procedures that required copious amounts of pure medicinal cocaine. As an adult he had regular incapacitating sinus attacks. Because of the deviated right septum, he could not breathe fully through his right nostril. This means he was predominately activating the more creative, artistic, nonverbal side of his brain. It is not surprising, then, that Kevin felt like an alien in his military family. He says he grew up in a world where the "status quo must be preserved at all cost." There were no emotional displays, positive or negative. Authority was respected. Secrets were kept. He could never understand why he was more introspective than his friends, and why he so often struggled with depression. "It was in my mid-teens that I began to realize how different I was from my contemporaries—so much more reflective and contemplative, and at the same time self-medicating with an abundance of alcohol and marijuana." But Kevin came alive on the stage. He performed throughout high school, was voted most talented boy in his senior class, and received a scholarship to study theater in college. "Only when I was high, performing, or training my body, was I free from depression's grip."

While Kevin was self-medicating his depression with alcohol and drugs and dancing professionally in New York City, his brother committed suicide. Kevin left New York, entered therapy, and began studying Yoga more seriously.

In Yogic terms, Kevin's suffering can be explained by an imbalance in his energy channels (*nadis*). As a left-nostril breather, Kevin was continually enhancing his lunar, cooling energy channels, the *ida nadis*, and had no balance with his solar, *pingala*, heating, energy channels, which, because of the way he was breathing, were mostly dormant. When he began studying Yoga in his thirties, he learned the importance of breathing on both the right and left sides of his body, balancing the ida and the pingala, the cooling and heating energies. To compensate for his still-deviated right septum, he began a regular practice of Right-Nostril Breathing, also known as Vitality-Stimulating Breath (*Surya Bheda*). "Twenty years of chronic depression lifted like a cloud," he says. Kevin feels that Right-Nostril Breathing would not have been effective if he were still drinking and had not gone through years of traditional psychotherapy. For Kevin, recovering from depression was a multipronged approach, but he believes that learning and practicing Right-Nostril Breathing was "the crowning touch."

Calming the Anxiety

We've been looking at the ways in which Yoga practice in general and pranayama breathing exercises in particular can balance the mood and relieve depression. But how, specifically, can pranayama soothe a person whose depression is characterized by anxiety?

Penny Smith and her daughter, both of whom you met in Chapter Two, suffer from bipolar disorder. They are among the 20 percent of manic-depressives who suffer from panic attacks. The first time Penny remembers having a major panic attack was in church. She was in an adult education class and everyone was taking turns reading aloud, an activity in which she had participated many times before. Just before her turn to read, her hands began to sweat and her heart began to race. When it was her turn at last, she could barely breathe. "I had to hold my breath while reading and thought I would pass out. That was my last time in that class." Within a few months, she was hospitalized for major depression.

After she was released, she was pushing Peggy, then two, on the playground swings, when she became unable to breathe. "My chest hurt, my hands were sweating, and I was sure that I would have a heart attack. No one else was around, and I was afraid I would die right there and my two-year-old would be alone on the playground." The panic attack lasted about ten minutes, and when it was over, she could barely walk the two blocks home. After that, she had many more panic attacks, and her doctor added Xanax, an antianxiety medication, to her regimen of antidepressants. As the anxiety grew worse and the panic attacks came more often, he kept increasing the dosage and her dependence on the drug grew.

Penny had been taking Xanax for a year when she began doing Yoga and pranayama breathing exercises. "I realized that when I felt an attack coming on, if I inhaled slowly for the count of four and blew the breath out through my mouth for the count of eight, that I could stop the attacks within a minute. I could also incorporate this breath almost any-where without anyone realizing that I was doing it." Following this practice, Penny has not had a panic attack for ten years and no longer takes Xanax. "I believe this is due to the fact that I incorporate various breathing techniques in my daily Yoga," she says. Penny practices Skull-Shining

Breath (Kapalabhati) before her postures, Ocean-Sounding Victory Breath (Ujjayi) during postures, and Alternate-Nostril Breathing with Retention afterward. "I am less stressed due to the Yoga, so I imagine that is another reason I no longer get them. I even made it through the death of my mother and my recent divorce without any attacks."

Penny's daughter was eight years old when she experienced her first panic attack. Peggy was enrolled in the children's program at Kripalu Center while Penny was attending a Yoga teachers' conference. When the children's program staff took the children for a walk after dinner, they encountered horses in the field in front of Kripalu. They took a shortcut back, which meant going under an electric fence surrounding the field. "Apparently, there was plenty of room to duck under, but the thought of it somehow caused panic in Peggy. After they got past the fence and back to the front of Kripalu, the kids decided to run partway up the hill. Peggy could not breathe or run. She had to sit down."

A week later, as Peggy was getting ready for bed, she was unable to breathe. "Her heart was racing and she looked very scared. I recognized it as a panic attack." Penny taught her to inhale through her nose for the slow count of four and blow out through her mouth for the count of eight. When Peggy was able to do this with her mother, there was an immediate improvement, but there were times when she felt too much panic and was unable to follow. At these times, Penny asked her to sing "Old MacDonald" as loud as she could. "You have to exhale longer than inhaling when you sing 'e-i-e-i-o,'" says Penny.

Yoga teacher and therapist Rami Katz has adapted Kundalini Yoga breathing and Yoga exercises along with other healing modalities in her work with individuals and groups at Cottonwood de Tucson, a residential treatment center in Arizona. She works with people suffering from anxiety and depression, eating disorders, PTSD, alcoholism, and other addictions, in groups, individually, and in classes. Since many of her clients have trouble breathing deeply—often the people she works with have developed a shallow, chest breathing due to anxiety-based depression, cigarette smoking, or asthma—she uses kinesthetic techniques to help them feel and understand the difference between their customary breathing patterns and the potential of deep diaphragmatic breathing. "Sometimes with people who smoke and use smoking as a way of feeling better, deep breathing is very difficult because it makes them feel dizzy.

Many people who aren't used to deep breathing, particularly people who are depressed, can feel very constricted in their chest and tight, and when they try to breathe deeply, they feel as though they're suffocating."

If you have poor breathing habits, it may be easier for you, like Rami's clients, to begin slowly. You may feel more relaxed if you begin on your back. With one hand on your belly and the other on your chest, you can more easily feel the movement of breath simply by paying attention to the rise and fall of your hands. "By concentrating on the hands and dividing the breath into parts," Rami says, "even people with asthma and other respiratory problems can learn to breathe fully and deeply." When deep diaphragmatic breathing is uncomfortable, Rami will sometimes use chanting, even with people who are unfamiliar with Eastern practices. One such client, who was extremely anxious, found relief from his anxiety by repeatedly chanting "Ong." In order to chant a mantra like "Ong" or "Om" or "Sat Nam," you first have to take a deep inhalation, thereby expanding the lungs. To make the sound, you must exhale slowly. Mantra chanting can physically open the lobes of the lungs.

Pranayama breathing may be the practice that enabled Cindy, a successful corporate lawyer working for a large firm in Tucson, to finally carry a pregnancy to birth. She and her husband had tried to have children for years, and at thirty-eight, her biological clock was ticking away. She had suffered through two miscarriages, and her doctors had told her that there were no physiological reasons why she could not conceive and bear a child. After her second miscarriage last year, her grief seemed endless, and she felt that her ability to do her job was suffering. Her gynecologist suggested that her level of anxiety might be a factor contributing to her inability to have a baby. She referred Cindy to a psychologist, who diagnosed the problem as an anxiety-based depression. Cindy had been taking medication for several months, had cut back her hours at the law firm, and was already feeling better when she began to practice Yoga. Still, I noticed rigidity in her upper body, a kind of armoring that kept her breath shallow and her speech rapid and breathy. Sometimes, after class, she talked to me about something that was bothering her, like her annoyance with the sound of the pounding treadmill that was occasionally in use in the room over the Yoga studio at the Tucson Racquet Club. Often, she spoke so quickly that she gasped for breath at the end of her speech.

I encouraged Cindy to practice Yogic Three-Part Breathing (Dirga Pranayama), described in the Yoga Experience in Chapter Two, off the Yoga mat whenever she was feeling anxious or upset, and to add to that the Ocean-Sounding Victory Breath (Ujjayi). A week later, she told me that she had been involved in a fender-bender, while pulling out of a parking space, in which she had scraped the paint off the door of her sports car. "I immediately began to practice Yogic Three-Part Breathing, and though I was annoyed with myself, I didn't get upset the way I usually do." Cindy practiced Yogic Three-Part Breath and Ocean-Sounding Victory Breath at home, and two months later, she told me she was pregnant. She continued practicing Yoga through her pregnancy, enrolling in a prenatal class, and seven months later, she gave birth to her first child.

"Breathing," says Yoga physiologist David Coulter, Ph.D., "is one of the most remarkable functions of anatomy and physiology. It is the only biological activity which can be brought under full conscious control and yet functions semiautomatically twenty-four hours a day."[11] If you do nothing else but commit to learning pranayama breathing, you will bring not only your breath under conscious control, but also your emotions. This doesn't mean you will repress your feelings, but rather you will begin to witness and more ably manage them.

Stoking the Fire

We have mostly been talking about Yogic Breathing that calms the fire, but what if you need to flame the fire in your belly? What if, like the poet Danna Faulds, you have suffered from a dysthymic depression for most of your life? Take heart—there are specific Yogic breathing exercises that can help you, too. Depressed on and off through much of her childhood, Danna received the message early on that it wasn't safe to be who she was. "I was raised in a strict Episcopal church where the message 'Lord I'm not worthy so much as to gather up the crumbs under thy table' was one I took in deeply—one could say cellularly." She feels she may have learned depression as a way of dealing with the world from her mother. Danna has been practicing Kripalu Yoga for nineteen years, and though she is not completely free of symptoms, her episodes of depression are now shorter and less intense. Danna has come to recognize the signs of an encroaching depression and can begin to adjust her pranayama breathing practice to manage her symptoms better than she could in the past.

What she notices first is a groping for words. "I'm a writer, and I literally lose words that I know. It's as if I'm standing on one side of a synapse, peering to the other side. There's a word there—the very word I want for a poem I'm writing—but I can't reach it. It remains there, dancing, just beyond my ability to grasp it. It's a very frustrating experience, and it invariably signals the onset of depression." Along with "losing words," Danna notices that she becomes more self-judgmental and harsh than she usually is. Her negative self-talk evokes a sense of worthlessness. "I'll write a perfectly decent poem and feel like it's nothing, worse than nothing. I'm worse than nothing."

Danna is more likely now to catch the early warning signs—the inability to find the words she wants and the first stirrings of self-judgment—and isn't blindsided by depression. "I know to be very watchful, and to refuse to give in to the self-judgments. I know to take good care of myself." For Danna, increasing her prana by getting outdoors, taking long walks, and riding her bike can help. And she considers her pranayama breathing practice one of her most effective tools.

When Danna notices depressive symptoms, she does a lengthy breathing practice after her posture session. Danna works carefully with her mood and the timing of her practice. She knows from experience that overdoing her pranayama breathing exercises is not beneficial and can actually be harmful. Too much Skull-Shining Breath (Kapalabhati), for example, can result in feelings of intense agitation. This is a good sign of the effectiveness of her breathing practice for overcoming depression. In the same way, psychopharmacologists recognize that a particular antidepressant is effective if in too high a dose it triggers anxiety or mania. Yes, you can overdose on pranayama breathing exercises just as you can overdose on antidepressant medication, which is why it's important to learn and practice the more energizing techniques with a qualified teacher.

Danna knows, having had direct experience of the anxiety-producing effects of practicing too much Skull-Shining Breath, to moderate her breathing session. When she is feeling anxious, rather than long rounds of energizing breathing exercises, she practices more soothing, balancing breathing exercises. "I've found that rhythmic deep breathing, and especially Alternate-Nostril Breathing (Nadi Sodhana), can be very nurturing, and even allow me to be 'outside' of the depression for a time."

Rama Jyoti Vernon feels so strongly about the risks of the more energizing breathing exercises that she no longer includes the more vigorous techniques like Skull-Shining Breath and Bellows Breath in her teacher-training courses. Rama teaches pranayama breathing almost exclusively within the practice of the postures, instead of in separate breathing sessions like those Danna, Penny, and others practice. Rather than the more energizing practices, Rama teaches Ocean-Sounding Victory Breath (Ujjayi) and Alternate-Nostril Breathing (Nadi Sodhana). Whether a student has "too much fire" (anxiety or mania) "or not enough" (dysthymia, major depression), breathing in this way, she says, "neutralizes the energy."

However, for those who are out of balance and suffering from dysthymia, like Danna, I would not be so cautious. Many Western teachers continue to teach the more fiery breathing techniques. In my own recovery from depression and in the work that I have done to support my students in moving out of their dark places, I find that the energizing techniques are an important element in the maintenance of a bright outlook. When I practice Skull-Shining or Bellows Breath, I pause to feel my energy. I often note a sense of expansion, as though my energy has enlarged beyond the limits of my physical body. These energizing practices give me a felt sense of a healing state that I believe is in part responsible for my recovery from depression and my continued well-being.

Pumping the Belly

In Skull-Shining Breath and Breath of Fire, a practice in the Kundalini tradition, a natural belly pumping occurs. In both cases, the breathing is rapid and the belly snaps back toward the spine on the exhalation and expands on the inhalation. According to a modern interpretation of ancient Yogic wisdom, the chakra located at the solar plexus, *manipura chakra,* is the center of self-esteem and identity. So when the belly is pumped vigorously in this way, you may be energizing your own personal power.

Many Yoga traditions teach a stomach-pumping exercise that heats and energizes the core of the body. In the Kripalu tradition, there is a stomach-pumping sequence called *Uddiyana Bandha* and *Agni Sara*, which literally means stomach lock with agitating fire. This is a sequence of stomach pumping with the breath held out, followed by Skull-Shining Breath. I practice this combination every day as an aid to digestion and elimination. Not only does my body feel energized after the practice, I also feel mentally brighter and more alert.

Marie, now a Yoga teacher in San Diego who has been practicing eight years, was feeling like "a highly stressed out small-business owner who just wanted a Mack truck to run over me and take me off the planet!" For depression, her teacher, Rama Berch, the founder of Svaroopa Yoga, recommended a hundred uddiyana bandhas daily. "Uddiyana Bandha helps with depression by increasing *udana* prana," says Rama Berch. Udana prana is "an upward-moving energy, which is the energy of happiness, laughter, and feeling 'up.'" Along with her daily routine of foundational poses, Marie practiced the bandhas every day. "After three months, the depression was gone. I could think about the business and not sink into a black hole." After that, she practiced Uddiyana Bandha only when she felt low. Last year, Marie finally quit the business she had come to loathe. "Looking back, had I maintained the daily practice of one hundred Uddiyana Bandhas for more than those first three months, maybe it wouldn't have taken me so long to make the final transition of selling the business and becoming a full-time Yoga teacher."

yoga experience

Pranayama Breathing Basics

1. It's important to have fresh air circulating in the room where you are practicing pranayama breathing exercises. Open a window, or go outside. Carrie, a graduate student in Philadelphia who has been subject to episodes of depression for most of her life, begins her practice outside no matter the weather. "The idea of just going outside and breathing a little will overcome the unexplainable resistance I have to doing Yoga by myself."

2. It is best to wait at least two hours after eating before practicing any pranayama.

3. Sit with the spine erect, just off the edge of a cushion, with legs crossed in Easy Pose or in Half-Lotus. You may also sit in Rock Pose Japanese-style on the knees, with the hips elevated by a meditation bench or a cushion. If none of these poses works for you, sit in a straight-backed chair. Begin with the palms open on the knees.

Balancing, Calming Breaths

Don't forget Yogic Three-Part Breath (Dirga), an excellent calming breath described in the Yoga Experience in Chapter Two. You can enhance your practice of this breath with Ocean-Sounding Victory Breath, described below. You can practice both breaths seated on a cushion or while you are moving into, holding, or releasing postures.

Ocean-Sounding Victory Breath (Ujjayi)

This breath can be practiced in a seated position as above, or lying down. Once you learn Ujjayi, practice it throughout your posture sequence, bringing a fresh supply of oxygen to the cells. To begin, inhale through your nostrils with a slight constriction of your throat, making a snoring sound. Maintain the slight snoring sound on the exhalation, and imagine that you are actually breathing from the back of your throat. I like to think of the sound as a wave gently rolling across pebbles. Breathe slowly, expanding the belly, the rib cage, and the upper chest. As you exhale, pull the abdomen in and up to empty your lungs completely. Let the breath be like a lullaby to yourself.

Purifying Breath—Alternate-Nostril Breathing (Nadi Sodhana)

The ancient Yogins believed that there were 72,000 (some traditions give a different number) tubelike channels traveling through the body called *nadis*. Some contemporary Yogins correlate the nadis to the nerves, while others think of the network of nadis in purely spiritual terms. Either way, Yogins believe it is important to keep as many nadis open as possible, so that the maximum prana may be conducted through the body. We begin Nadi Sodhana by balancing the nadis on the left side of the body with the nadis on the right. Yogins believe that there are three main conductors: First, there is the *ida,* which conducts energy through the left nostril, and the *pingala*, which conducts energy through

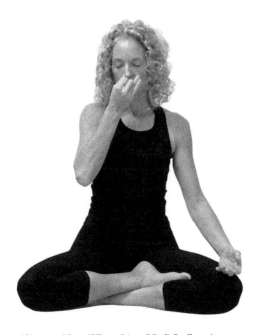

Alternate-Nostril Breathing (Nadi Sodhana)

the right nostril. These two main conductors weave around the central axial nadi, the *sushumna*, which travels the length of the spine, ending at the crown chakra (*sahasrara*). In some traditions, it is believed that the ida and pingala cross each other at the chakras, forming a ladder of energy to the sixth chakra (*ajna*) at the brow point. We start with Nadi Sodhana so that both nostrils are free and clear and the left and right sides of the body and brain are functioning in balance.

Sit with the spine erect. Make a fist of your right hand. Next, release the thumb and the third and fourth fingers, leaving the index and middle fingers against your palm. Place the thumb against your right nostril and slowly inhale through your left. Close off the left nostril with the fourth and little fingers of your right hand and hold the breath for one or two seconds. Then release your thumb and slowly exhale through your right. Inhale through your right, then close off the right nostril, pause, then exhale through your left. Repeat. Keep the inhalation even with the exhalation. Do five rounds to begin, ending by exhaling through your left nostril.

Sit with the eyes closed and notice how you are feeling. Are you feeling calmer? More alert? Nadi Sodhana may be practiced as a way to center yourself before Yoga asanas, before meditation, or any time you would like to enhance your feeling of equanimity.

Retention (Kumbhaka)

When you are comfortable and steady in your practice of Yogic Three-Part Breath (Dirga), Ocean-Sounding Victory Breath (Ujjayi), and Purifying Alternate-Nostril Breathing (Nadi Sodhana), you may begin to hold the breath at the top of the inhalation, initially for just a short time, perhaps for a count of four. You might also experiment with lengthening the exhalation and pausing briefly before inhaling again. A good beginning ratio is: four counts in; hold the breath in for four counts; exhale for six counts; hold the breath out for two counts. Shirley Telles and her colleagues at the Vivekanandra Kendra have studied the effect of breath retention. Their research indicates that short breath retention (four to six counts) energizes the body, while longer holding of the breath (more than six to maximum capacity) seems to calm the body. With short retention, there is "a significant increase [52 percent] in oxygen consumption and metabolic rate, compared to the pre-pranayamic baseline period of breathing. In contrast, the long kumbhak [retention] pranayamic breathing caused a statistically significant lowering [19 percent] of the oxygen consumption and metabolic rate."[12]

After you have learned and practiced the calming breathing exercises and are comfortable with them, you may experiment with short breath retention between each breath. When practicing the energizing breathing exercises, you may wish to experiment with a longer holding of the breath after you've completed a full round of the exercise. Your practice of retention will be enhanced by learning the locks from a qualified teacher.

Bee Breath (Brahmari)

This breathing practice slows down the exhalation and has a calming effect on the entire nervous system. In India, it is often recommended for women in labor. Sit in a comfortable position with the spine erect. Constrict the glottis at the back of your throat and inhale through the nostrils. If you wish, as you inhale, practice making a high-pitched buzzing sound that comes from the back of your throat. The emphasis

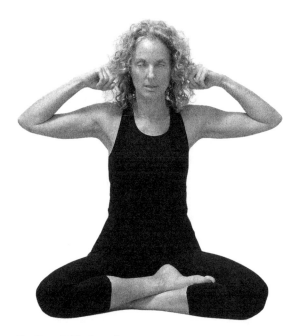

Bee Breath (Brahmari)

of this practice is on the exhalation. Exhale slowly through the nostrils, making a deep buzzing sound in your throat like a bee. Let your tongue vibrate lightly against the roof of your mouth. Practice this breath ten to twenty times, taking resting breaths in between as needed. Notice your energy. As you become more comfortable with the breath, you may practice the locks, while holding the breath out between rounds. You may also, with your index fingers, push your earlobes up and press them against the opening to your ear canal, blocking the sound outside your body.

Fanning the Fire

Study the activating breaths with a qualified teacher, but only after you have established a strong practice of the balancing, calming pranayama breathing exercises described earlier.

Please do not practice these breathing exercises if you are pregnant, menstruating, or have unmedicated high blood pressure. If you suffer from bipolar disorder, please consult with your psychiatrist before practicing. Any of these energizing breaths could trigger a manic episode.

Skull Shining (Kapalabhati)

Though it is a breathing exercise, Kapalabhati is not technically a pranayama. Rather, it is a *kriya* (complete purifying action), which cleanses not only the nasal passages but the entire system, flooding the body with prana. Kriyas include many kinds of complete and cleansing actions that have little to do with the breath. But you don't need to be concerned about the difference between a pranayama and a kriya. Just enjoy the practice. Skull-Shining Breath is a wonderful way to wake up the dormant prana if you are feeling depressed.

Sit with the spine erect. Exhale forcefully through both nostrils while snapping the belly back toward the spine. The inhalations are so passive that you barely notice them. Simply receive the breath. Begin with twenty repetitions. As you become more proficient, you can increase the speed and number of repetitions.

Skull Shining with Retention (Kapalabhati with Kumbhaka)

This practice should be attempted only after you are comfortable with Ocean-Sounding Victory Breath (Ujjayi), Yogic Three-Part Breath

(Dirga), Alternate-Nostril Breathing (Nadhi Sodhana), and Skull-Shining Breath (Kapalabhati). Please work with a teacher when learning the locks (bandhas).*

After the final exhalation in your round of kapalabhati, inhale and hold the breath in for a count of five, then lean forward and exhale all the breath in your lungs through the mouth. With the breath held out, lift your spine to a straight position as you lift the pelvic floor, using the root lock (*mula bandha*). Next, draw your navel back and up toward the spine. This movement of navel to spine is called the stomach lock (*uddiyana bandha*). You may also drop your chin toward your chest as you raise your chest to meet your chin. This movement, called the throat lock (*jalandhara bandha*), stimulates the thyroid and parathyroid glands at your throat chakra (*vishuddha*). Hold the breath out for a count of five to ten, using all three locks if you are comfortable with them. When you need to inhale, release the locks, beginning first with the root lock, next the stomach lock, then the throat lock. Lift your head so that your chin is again parallel to the floor and breathe in, filling your lungs to two-thirds capacity. Hold the breath for five to ten counts. Then slowly release the breath with a whistle. Sit for a moment and observe the energy circulating through your body. You may repeat this sequence up to three times.

Alternate-Nostril Skull Shining (Kapalabhati)

Sit as above. Bring your right hand into the position you used for Alternate-Nostril Breathing (Nadhi Sodhana). Using your right hand, place the thumb over the right nostril while exhaling forcefully through the left and snapping the belly back, then place the fourth and little fingers of your right hand over your left nostril while exhaling through the right nostril and snapping the belly back. Take little sips of breath through both nostrils between exhalations. Complete your round of breathing by exhaling through the left nostril. After your round of Alternate-Nostril Skull-Shining Breath, you may practice breath retention (kumbhaka) and expulsion, using the locks as above.

---

*I haven't changed my mind about the importance of studying the locks (bandhas) with a teacher, but you will find them here, because, when used with some of the pranayama breathing exercises, I have found them to be beneficial in my own and my students' recovery, particularly from dysthymic depression.

Breath of Fire

Sit with the spine erect. Take forceful inhalations and exhalations of even lengths, snapping the belly back toward the spine on the exhalations. You can use this breath alone or you may try it when you are holding a posture.

Mountain Breath

Sit with the spine erect, arms out alongside your body, fingertips touching the floor. Slowly inhale the arms out to your sides and up over your head. Interlace your fingers, index fingers extended. Hold the breath for as long as you can while lifting up the pelvic floor (mula bandha or root lock). When you can't hold the breath any longer, slowly release it as your arms float down to the starting position. (If you feel too much energy, take a long, slow breath in and out through your nostrils.) Repeat, and this time, in addition to lifting the pelvic floor, draw your navel back toward your spine as you hold the breath (uddiyana bandha or stomach

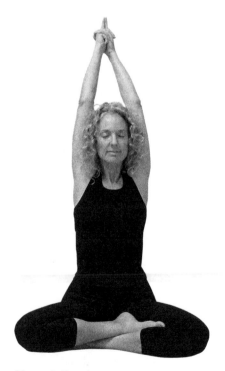

Mountain Breath

lock). Slowly release. Repeat, and this time, in addition to the root lock and the stomach lock, drop your chin to your chest as you hold the breath (jalandhara bandha or throat lock). Slowly release. Repeat. Use all three locks while holding the breath and pressing your tongue to the soft palate at the roof of your mouth. Draw your eyes up behind their lids. Hold the breath. Slowly release. Repeat, using all three locks. Then, while holding the breath and continuing to hold the root and stomach locks, release the throat lock, lifting your chin so that it is parallel to the floor, and open your hands so that your arms are shoulder-width apart with your palms facing each other. As you hold your breath, imagine energy pouring through your chakras. Slowly release. Sit and receive the energy.

Bellows Breath (Bhastrika)

This breath is especially good for dysthymia, because the vagus nerve is stimulated, which is a known treatment for depression. There is also a probable release of the "feel-good" hormones oxytocin and prolactin.

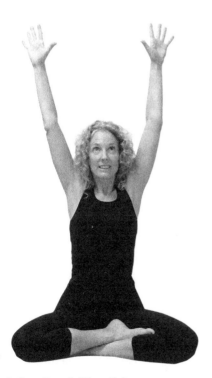

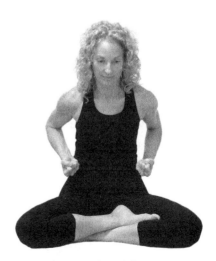

Bellows Breath (Bhastrika):
Inhale your arms up

Bellows Breath (Bhastrika):
Exhale vigorously

The subjective experience is one of mild elation followed by a feeling of relaxation. Various Yoga traditions teach Bellows Breath differently. It is similar to Skull-Shining Breath, but the inhalation is deep and forceful, equal to the exhalation, and is usually done at a slower pace. It can be practiced with or without the arm movements. This is how I lead it.

Sit with your spine erect, either with the support of a meditation bench or a pillow propped between your thighs. If this is uncomfortable, you may choose another seated position like Half-Lotus, or you may sit in an armless chair with your spine straight. Bend your elbows and make fists with your hands with the upper arms hugging the torso. Take a normal natural breath in and out. As you inhale through the nostrils, send your arms straight up over your head, with great force as you open your palms to face outward, spreading your fingers wide. Exhale with great force through the nostrils as you bring your arms back to the starting position, again making fists with your hands. Do this at a moderate pace twenty times, then rest for thirty seconds. Practice two more rounds of twenty each, pausing for at least thirty seconds between rounds. When you've completed the practice, sit for several moments, observing the effects. Notice your mood. As you become more experienced with the practice, you can add breath retention and the locks between rounds.

Right-Nostril Vitality Breath (Surya Bheda)

Sit in a comfortable position with your spine straight. As in Alternate-Nostril Breathing, make a fist of your right hand. Next, release the thumb and the third and fourth fingers, keeping the index finger and middle finger folded toward your palm. Close off the left nostril with the fourth and little fingers of your right hand and breathe in through your right nostril. Close off both nostrils and hold the breath for four counts. While holding the breath, drop the chin into throat lock (jalandhara bandha), then lift the pelvic floor for the root lock (mula bandha). Then release the locks—first the root lock, then the throat lock—close your right nostril with your thumb, and exhale through your left nostril. Practice up to ten rounds. As you become more experienced with the breath, you can increase the length of the retention. After your practice, close your eyes and notice your energy. If you feel too "bright," practice a few rounds of Alternate-Nostril Breathing to bring you back into balance.

Uddiyana Bandha and Agni Sara

This breathing exercise combines several techniques you have already learned. It is excellent to practice in the morning before breakfast, as it facilitates digestion and elimination. It should not be practiced if you suffer from irritable bowel syndrome or any other inflammation of the digestive or intestinal tract. Do not practice this exercise if you are menstruating or pregnant.

To begin, stand with the feet a comfortable distance apart and inhale, raising the arms over your head. Exhale fully through the mouth and bring the hands to the knees with the back and elbows straight. With the breath held out, draw the navel back and up toward the spine, then roll the abdomen up and back in a circular motion until you need to breathe again (*nauli*). Inhale back to standing and practice twenty rounds of Skull-Shining Breath, either through both nostrils or, if you

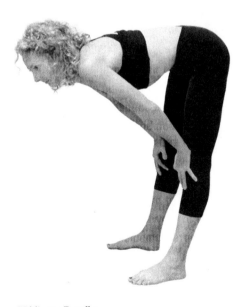

Uddiyana Bandha

are comfortable, through alternate nostrils. Repeat the entire sequence two more times. Close your eyes and notice your energy. You may want to place your hands on your belly to feel the energy you've generated at the core of your body.

Breath of Joy

Stand with the feet a comfortable distance apart and your arms at your sides. Inhale one-third capacity through your nostrils and swing your arms up to shoulder level in front of you. Inhale to two-thirds capacity and stretch your arms out to the sides. Inhale to full capacity and swing your arms up over your head. As you exhale through your mouth, lean forward and stretch your arms out to the sides and slightly behind you. Repeat four more times. Return to standing. Close your eyes and experience the effects.

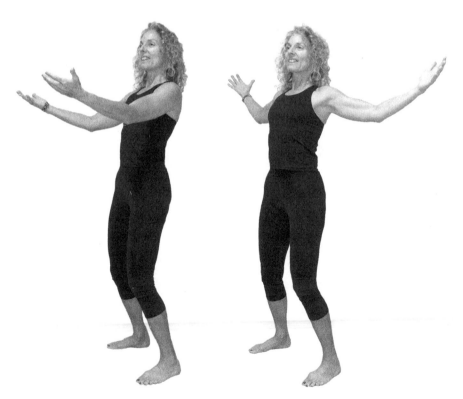

Breath of Joy: Inhale to 1/3 capacity   *Breath of Joy: Inhale to 2/3 capacity*

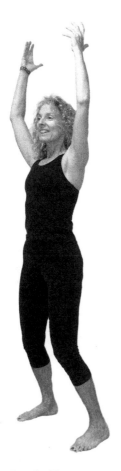
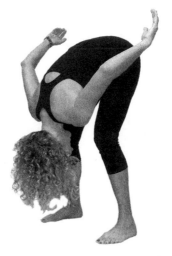
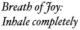

Breath of Joy:
Inhale completely

Breath of Joy:
Exhale vigorously

Power Hara

This standing energizing breath adds a twist, which can feel very good for a stiff spine. Stand with your feet wider than hip-width apart and bring your hands to your shoulders with your elbows pointed out like chicken wings. Inhale, filling your lungs halfway, and twist to the left. Inhale fully and twist to the right. Then extend your right arm forcefully to the left as you twist to the left, exhaling through your mouth with a "ha" sound. Extend your left arm forcefully to the right as you twist to

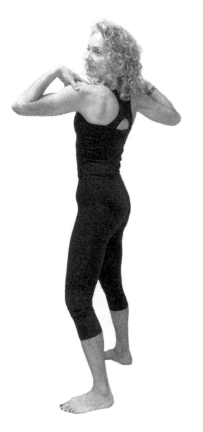

Power Hara: Inhale twist

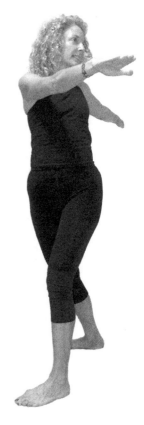

Power Hara: Exhale extend

the right, exhaling again through your mouth with a "ha" sound. Practice ten full rounds. Release, close your eyes, and feel your awakened energy.

art of living—
breathing that heals

I want to unfold.
Let no place in me hold itself closed,
for where I am closed, I am false.
I want to stay clear in your sight.

—RANIER MARIA RILKE, from "I'm so alone in the world"[1]

In 1999, while researching an article about Yoga and depression for *Yoga Journal* magazine, I came across numerous studies done by the National Institute of Mental Health and Neurosciences in India, in which *Sudharshan Kriya* (SK), a breathing practice taught around the world by the Art of Living Foundation, was found to have as high as a 73 percent recovery rate in the treatment of hospitalized patients suffering from major depression. The statistics were astounding. Time after time, in controlled studies, Sudharshan Kriya compared favorably to other treatments for depression, including antidepressant medications and electroconvulsive therapy (ECT). In India there is an "Attitude Toward Yoga" scale that is administered to patients entering such studies. Many of the hospitalized patients were disturbed to be in the "Yoga breathing group" and would have preferred to take medication. Yet these same people experienced a statistically significant recovery rate from depression despite their initial resistance to learning a Yoga technique.

In my interviews with Art of Living teachers and students, I encountered friendly, trusting people who seemed happier than most people I knew, even those who have done spiritual practice of one kind or another for a long time. They told me about their own personal healings, their recoveries from head injury, hypertension, coronary disease, and depression. They told me how much more energy they felt and how much happier they were in their relationships and with their lives. What they didn't tell me was how to practice Sudharshan Kriya. For that, I was told I would have to take the course with a qualified Art of Living teacher.

Chris Dale, a teacher from Australia, described SK this way: "a unique Vedic breathing meditation, using set breathing rhythms, which harmonize the rhythms of body, breath, mind, and emotions and take the practitioner deep into pure Being." According to the Art of Living teachers with whom I spoke, the technique washes away deep-rooted stresses, detoxifies the body, and powerfully balances the system at all levels. Later, in preparation for this book, I talked with psychopharmacologist and associate professor of clinical psychiatry at Columbia University Dr. Richard Brown, coauthor of *Stop Depression Now*, who explained in detail the known and hypothesized physiological actions involved in the pranayama breathing exercises and Sudharshan Kriya. I wanted to understand why, from a medical standpoint, this program, in controlled studies around the world, has shown such a high rate of success in the treatment of depression, anxiety disorders, attention deficit disorder, post-traumatic stress disorder (PTSD), and prevention of relapse in alcohol treatment.[2]

Why It Works

A recent study assessed the level of anxiety, anger, fear, and reactive behavior among juvenile offenders in Los Angeles before and after taking the Prison Smart Program, the cornerstone of which is the breathing practice Sudharshan Kriya. Seventy-two detained youth, ages thirteen to eighteen, most of whom were gang members with prior incarcerations for violent crimes, completed a one-week training program and practiced the breathing technique for eight weeks. Despite a change in warden during the eight-week period, high staff turnover, and understaffing, there was a significant decrease in anxiety at the conclusion of the eight weeks. Fights and temporary disciplinary removal were also significantly reduced.[3]

Perhaps the reduction in violence happens in part because of the release of anterior pituitary hormones—oxytocin, prolactin, and vasopressin—during the practice. Prolactin, vasopressin, and oxytocin share many similarities, including what has been called a "feel-good" effect. Oxytocin, the "cuddle hormone," influences the bonding and affection mothers feel for their infants and is a primary sexual arousal hormone. According to Richard Brown and his wife, psychiatrist Patricia Gerbarg, authors of a recent study on the possible effects of Sudharshan Kriya, "there is some evidence of low oxytocin levels in major depression."[4] Studies have shown that prolactin levels increase in depressed patients who are taught Sudharshan Kriya. Prolactin is the hormone that is released in electroconvulsive therapy (ECT), and is regarded to be, at least in part, responsible for ECT's mood-elevating effect. Additionally, vasopressin (also low in people suffering from depression) has been shown to increase dramatically after TM (Transcendental Meditation) practice, and, Richard Brown hypothesizes, after SK as well. Drs. Brown and Gerbarg suggest that the probable increased levels of oxytocin, vasopressin, and prolactin resulting from the practice of Sudharshan Kriya may in part explain the healing effect it seems to have on depression. This elevation of hormone levels may account for the dramatic change among imprisoned terrorists in India after taking the Art of Living Course.

One of the most striking service projects run by the Art of Living Foundation is the work they are doing with prisoners, teaching Sudharshan Kriya in jails and detention centers in India and the United States. One convicted terrorist in India, an al Qaeda leader in fact, refused bail twice so that he could take the advanced Art of Living Course. According to Dr. Brown, who talked to convicted terrorists in Indian jails during a trip to present a scientific paper at a conference in New Delhi, the inmates who have taken the course say they can never again imagine killing or doing violence to another human being. "The head warden at Beur Model, a prison in Patna, said that the practice of Sudharshan Kriya has had a dramatic effect on the level of aggression and tension in the prison. The prisoners and jailers now greet each other with great respect. According to the warden, the three most hardened criminals, multiple killers actually, had become model prisoners and were helping the other prisoners."

"From a Western perspective," says Art of Living research director Ronnie Newman, "Sudharshan Kriya balances brain and hormone function in depressed individuals, which can account for the dramatic recovery from depression. From an Eastern perspective, the technique works to eradicate depression by flooding the body with prana." As do other teachers and Yoga therapists, Sri Sri Ravi Shankar, who developed the technique based on ancient practices, feels that depression is the result of diminished prana. "When our bodies are lively with prana," says Sri Sri, "we feel alert, energetic and full of good humor. A lack of prana results in lethargy, dullness and poor enthusiasm."[5]

According to Sri Sri, during the practice of Sudharshan Kriya, "every cell becomes fully oxygenated and flooded with new life. Negative emotions that have been stored as toxins in the body are easily uprooted and flushed out. Tensions, frustrations and anger get released. Anxiety, depression and lethargy are washed away."[6]

We'll look at how the claim that SK eliminates physical and emotional toxins at the cellular level might be explained physiologically. But first, without giving a guideline for practice, which I am not trained to do, I'll try to be as clear as I can about what the technique entails.

The preparatory pranayama breathing exercises, which are practiced before doing SK, are similar to those found in other traditions. The first breathing exercise, called Three-Stage Breathing, is practiced to open up full lung capacity. It is similar in some ways to the Yogic Three-Part Breath (Dirga), discussed in Chapter Two. It utilizes Ocean-Sounding Victory Breath (Ujjayi), breath retention, and *mudras* (seals), which are specific positions for the hands. Three-Stage Breathing opens up the lung capacity to receive more prana while practicing SK. The Institute for Rehabilitation of the Government of Slovenia conducted an independent pilot study of Sudharshan Kriya that included Three-Stage Breathing as an adjunct treatment for multiple sclerosis. Breathing can be difficult for MS patients. The disorder affects the central nervous system and negatively impacts diaphragm functioning, thereby reducing oxygen consumption. After only five days of the breathing practices, the MS patients showed a significant improvement in lung capacity and oxygen consumption.

The next preparatory pranayama is the Bellows Breath (Bhastrika), taught in a way that is similar to the way it is taught in other traditions. After the pranayama breathing exercises and prior to the practice of Sudharshan Kriya, three rounds of "Aum" may be chanted.

Finally, one does Sudharshan Kriya, an organized pattern of varying breath rhythms. After taking the Art of Living Course, one can practice the breathing techniques at home. The at-home practice of pranayama breathing exercises plus SK takes about twenty minutes. It can be practiced twice a day, or, if you have a meditation practice, a once-a-day practice, followed by meditation, is sufficient. The home practice is an excellent foundation for meditation. "Sudharshan Kriya takes away a lot of the stresses in the body/mind complex that normally come up in meditation as fidgeting or a lot of thoughts in the mind," says Manhattan Art of Living teacher Annelies Richmond. "When you practice Sudharshan Kriya first, you begin your meditation from a clear, clean place." Richard Brown speculates that the frontal cortex, which is the area of the brain engaged in planning, anticipation, worry, and carrying out plans, is quieted by the practice. It seems logical, then, that meditation would begin from a calmer, more relaxed state. Meditators who practice Sudharshan Kriya before they sit to meditate say that their meditation practice is deeper. Likely they are experiencing what researchers have called Stage II experience in meditation, in which the breath rate decreases, alpha waves increase in the brain, indicating deep relaxation, and the meditator has a subjective experience of "transcending" the ordinary conscious state.

In addition to the daily home practice, Sri Sri Ravi Shankar recommends that Sudharshan Kriya be done once a week in a group with a teacher. In this context, the entire practice takes more than one hour.

The combination of pranayama breathing exercises calms the mind, yet leaves it in a state of emotional receptivity and mental alertness.

Three-Stage Breathing uses Ocean-Sounding Victory Breath (Ujjayi), which research has shown activates the body's parasympathetic response system. This calms the body's autonomic functions (involuntary, like heartbeat, breath, and digestion). At the same time, the vagus nerve is likely stimulated, which lowers heart rate as the blood pressure is slightly and temporarily increased. As the vagal tone is enhanced through continued practice, the effects of stress on the heart are reduced. The subjective state is a feeling of calm alertness. According to Richard Brown, this is a highly focused, "vigilant" state often found in animals when they are aware of a predator or combatant. "What that translates into in an animal," he says, "is that the animal is much more resilient to stress. There is a greater range of activity in the sympathetic system, so if the animal is stressed and it needs to fight or flee, it has more reserves to do that. At the same time, the parasympathetic system is recharging the animal."

Chanting "Aum" has been shown to decrease metabolism and heart rate while increasing peripheral vascular resistance, thereby strengthening the vascular system. The result is that we feel brighter and more alert "in the context of physiological relaxation."[7] According to Dr. Dharma Singh Khalsa, the vibratory effect of mantra chanting has "a pronounced effect on our two most sensitive systems: the neurological and the endocrine systems."[8] Chanting, according to Dr. Khalsa and others, can improve immune functioning and increase brain hemispheric balance. Cynthia Kemp Scherer, a flower essence researcher and practitioner and author of the book *The Art & Technique of Using Flower Essences*, told me that she began a chanting practice many years ago, after treating a man suffering from an anxiety-based depression. One day, as she read his pulses, she found that he was calmer and more serene than he had been previously. When she questioned him, it turned out that he had begun chanting regularly with a local Yoga group.

Sudharshan Kriya itself is an alternating series of breathing patterns that Richard Brown and Patricia Gerbarg believe, based on studies of other techniques that share attributes with SK, stimulates the vagus nerve. A recent study used vagal nerve stimulation (VNS) therapy to treat patients suffering from severe depression who had failed to respond to an average of sixteen depression and mood treatments. According to Cyberonics, the company that developed the vagal nerve stimulation device, after three months of VNS, 40 percent of these 43 patients showed a 50 percent or greater improvement in depressive symptoms, and 21 percent achieved remission. Those who completed at least one year of VNS therapy had an even better remission rate. However, VNS therapy is invasive. The device is surgically implanted in the chest and has unwanted side effects. Not only does the device stimulate the brain through the vagus nerve, but it also stimulates the diaphragm, which affects the voice. "VNS therapy may make people a little more prone to asthma," says Richard Brown, "because it slightly constricts the airways. It may also increase acid secretion in the stomach, so people with the device implanted may be a little more prone to ulcers. And it costs $25,000." According to both Richard Brown and Art of Living's Ronnie Newman, Sudharshan Kriya is a natural way to achieve a similar effect without the side effects. In fact, it actually has a higher success rate than VNS therapy for achieving remission from the symptoms of depression.

Sudharshan Kriya may also produce an "edge of sleep" state, from which repressed memories and feelings may emerge. However, as Ronnie Newman points out, the process of release happens without cognition of the traumatic memory. In other words, says Newman, "Sudharshan Kriya is traditionally understood to release the biochemical toxins from the original traumatizing experience, saving the practitioner from having to reexperience the event."

Although there have been a number of studies showing the psychiatric effects of Sudharshan Kriya, there has not yet been work that analyzes precisely what happens in the body when a person practices SK. "However," hypothesizes Richard Brown, "the data from mechanical hyperventilation [studies] and the data from the vagal nerve stimulation [studies] give us a general idea of what this breathing is doing. I think the rhythm of the breathing adds an extra dimension that no one has studied."

In an interview with the *India Times*, Brown postulated the overall healing effects this way: "The breathing activates the vagus nerve that connects with the diaphragm and some of the organs, including the heart and the brain. As a result of this stimulation, messages are sent along three different pathways that tell the body to shut off areas of worry while awakening areas that control feelings of happiness in the brain. So, one pathway is created that leads up to the frontal cortex of the brain and starts shutting down areas controlling excess worries and depressions. Another pathway shuts off anxiety-producing parts of the brain stem and a third wakes up the limbic system, which controls positive emotions."[9]

Measuring the Immeasurable

Janael McQueen, director of teacher training for the Art of Living Foundation, has been practicing SK for eighteen years and, despite sharing the obstacles that most of us face on a regular basis, seems to walk with a light step. When I met her, she reminded me of what, in my search for scientific evidence, I might be overlooking. Was I behaving like those good neoscientists, Descartes and his seventeenth-century cronies, who ushered in the scientific Age of Enlightenment, discarding all that could not be proven? Might it be possible that research data and scientific speculation can actually limit our understanding of ancient techniques? I think so. When applying a Western medical model, we have to ask ourselves what is being missed on both a physiological and spiritual level when we break Yogic practices down into a clear relation between cause and effect. The benefits of a particular practice can be so much greater than one measured effect. Janael believes that when we are too analytic in our approach to understanding how Sudharshan Kriya works, we risk losing "the magic," and I agree. When we measure a particular effect of a technique on heart rate, let's say, we are not only ignoring a vast array of other physiological changes, but the subjective experience, the pleasure of the practice, goes unrecorded. As I began to study the scientific data that Richard Brown and his wife, psychiatrist Patricia Gerberg, had accumulated on the possible physiological explanations of why the SK technique works, even the research director for the Art of Living Foundation, Ronnie Newman, reminded me that when examining a technique, it's important to stay open to what is not being tested, to what is immeasurable.

Making a Difference

Annelies Richmond has been practicing Sudharshan Kriya for three and a half years. As a ballet dancer with the Metropolitan Opera, she has a heightened awareness about how Sudharshan Kriya affects her body. She says practicing SK helps relax her muscles by releasing the lactic acid that builds when she dances. "Sometimes, when I do Sudharshan Kriya, my spine will adjust itself." She feels more even and grounded, she says. "The longer I practice SK, the more unshakable I feel. After a few months of practicing, I noticed that when an upsetting event happened, I could watch it without becoming upset myself." The stage fright that used to plague her before a performance is gone. "It's so much more enjoyable to prepare and to perform without the nervousness."

Annelies has taught the Course to a number of people suffering from depression and anxiety. "A lot of my students have been stuck in a cycle of negative thinking for years. It's beautiful for me to see how Sudharshan Kriya and the Course breaks that." The students report back that they are sleeping much more soundly. One of her students, a graduate student at Columbia, had tremendous anxiety accompanied by a panic disorder that was disrupting his life. "When he arrived for the Course, he looked like a ghost—his face was completely white and he couldn't smile. After the first Kriya, his face was transformed—there was color in his cheeks, his eyes were bright, and he was smiling." According to Annelies, he practices SK twice a day now, and his panic attacks have disappeared.

Frank, a forty-seven-year-old computer network administrator in Baltimore, Maryland, says he was depressed for the first forty years of his life. In the course of his treatment, he'd taken antidepressants, had individual and group therapy, tried an outpatient hospital program, and self-medicated on drugs. He also traveled the alternative route—acupuncture, nutritional therapy, and Rolfing. "Nothing made a dent," he says. When he enrolled in the Art of Living Course in 1989, he did so because of his interest in pranayama breathing, not expecting to find relief from his depressive symptoms. "On the very first night of the course, I went grocery shopping, and as I walked through the store, I could feel that something had already begun changing." By the end of the course, "I saw the light at the end of the tunnel." Frank's progress has been steady, he says. "This disarmingly simple process has turned my life around."

Octavio was a well-respected orthodontist and university professor in Chile when he began suffering a series of physical symptoms that incapacitated him. His body trembled to such an extent that he couldn't use the tools of his profession. For three years, his life was a nightmare of professional setbacks and family problems caused by symptoms that, despite consultations with medical specialists all over the world, seemed to have no physical basis. Because of his prominent position in his community, he was reluctant to seek treatment from a mental health professional, but he believes now that he was suffering from a severe psychiatric illness, most likely depression. Not only was he unable to function in his work, but his family life became intolerable. He could not abide the normal voices of his children, and they were sent to live in California with his sister. Eventually his wife left him, too, and went to be with their daughters. After three years of worsening symptoms, he sold his practice, resigned from his university teaching position, and returned to the United States, where he had done his graduate training seventeen years earlier. Once resettled with his family in Colorado, he began exploring alternative medicine and healing practices like Reiki. Still, though, the days when he was unable to get out of bed in the morning outnumbered the days when he could. In 1995, he took the Art of Living Course and began to feel an immediate change for the better. He practiced regularly, and in the first few months, he began having more good days than bad ones.

Today, Octavio has been an Art of Living Teacher for five years, offering courses in South America. In one South American city, when a well-known physician's wife with chronic fatigue syndrome began to feel better after taking the course, many physicians and their spouses followed suit. Octavio says that teaching the Art of Living Course is the most gratifying work he has ever done. After seeing the changes in her husband, his wife took the Course, and now his entire family practices Sudharshan Kriya. His colleagues, where he now teaches high school biology, marvel at his positive attitude and the close relationships he has with many of his students. "I tell them I have seen the dark side, and I choose to practice a technique that illuminates my life."

The Guru Question

In Chapter Ten, we will explore the benefits and the potential pitfalls of a devotional path if you are suffering from depression, whether your devotion is through a beloved teacher or, more directly, to God. It is a question to be reckoned with if you are involved in a daily Yoga practice, no matter with what religious faith you are or are not affiliated. Eventually you may find that the practices you love were transmitted to your teacher through her teacher or guru. And you may be drawn to meet and study with that teacher, to experience for yourself the connection you may feel in that teacher's presence.

In 1999, I learned that the kindhearted Art of Living teachers I was talking with were all devotees of Sri Sri Ravi Shankar. Having witnessed too many spiritual teachers tumble off the pedestal their devotees had constructed, I had reservations about stepping onto a path where another Guru was involved. Then I began to hear that these devotee/ teachers were offering free special health courses in prisons, detention centers, and hospitals, and that many free courses were offered in New York City for those suffering the aftermath of the terrorist attacks on September 11, 2001. These teachers believed so passionately in what they were doing that they were willing to offer their time and service to those in need, without thought of remuneration. The generosity of the Art of Living teachers I met, and my desire to come from a place of experience with the technique when I wrote this chapter, finally inspired me to take the course in 2002.

Participants in the Art of Living Course sometimes ask questions about where Sudharshan Kriya comes from and who developed it, but the technique and philosophical teachings are delivered without much talk about a guru. "We don't hide the fact that Sri Sri Ravi Shankar is the custodian of this knowledge," says Ronnie Newman, "and then if people are interested, they are welcome to join the mainstream of Art of Living, to come to *satsanga* and develop a relationship with Sri Sri. But not only do we feel that it's not necessary to have any kind of relationship with the guru, it's not even encouraged. We simply want to provide people with the capacity to heal. Depending on where they are in their own personal journey, they can either take advantage of developing a relationship with Sri Sri or not."

According to Janael McQueen, Sri Sri Ravi Shankar is a teacher who avoids making decisions for his students. When asked by an interviewer about the meaning of life, Sri Sri said, "This is better you find out for yourself. Don't ask the meaning from me. It's like asking me to chew your candy for you."[10] Though for years, devoted as she was, Janael asked Sri Sri for a Sanskrit name, he would never give her one. There is no formal initiation process as there is in some other traditions; Sanskrit names are not necessarily bestowed upon the faithful. People travel to see Sri Sri Ravi Shankar from all over the world for reasons other than that they are formal disciples. Some say they feel healed by the power of his presence; others are uplifted by the teachings; still others are unaffected.

Suzanne is a Sudharshan Kriya practitioner who has remained unaffected. She is a forty-year-old art director in Manhattan with a family history of depression and alcoholism, who dates her depression (dysthymia with anxiety and episodes of major depression) to the age of twelve. At that time, Suzanne's mother became seriously ill and Suzanne took over her mother's caretaking role in the family. Suzanne has taken the Art of Living Course several times and feels that, as a result, she is less anxious and depressed. "I'm a little skeptical," she says. "Art of Living people often tell me that when you're in Sri Sri Ravi Shankar's presence, you feel the energy. I do think he's a great teacher who has done a tremendous amount of good, but personally, I don't feel his energy." Still others, like Annelies Richmond, feel uplifted in the presence of the man they consider to be their teacher. "If you have any problems and questions, when you're in Sri Sri's presence, they slip away. You feel happy and at ease around him."

Richard Brown, who has maintained a Zen martial arts practice for many years, was skeptical at first. For two years, he referred patients to the Course without taking it himself. Over the years of his practice, he says he has met a lot of pseudogurus and enlightened teachers. "One thing I've learned, doing years of martial arts and Zen and psychiatry, is that you can get an idea of a person's inner mind, the inner self, and the person's intentions by the things he does—it's like you see the wind blowing by seeing the leaves move." When Richard Brown finally took the Course, he realized that "whoever had created this course had very deep knowledge." One of his frustrations as a martial arts practitioner was that very few people make great progress. "Maybe one in a thousand," he says. When he took the Art of Living Course, he knew he had found something that would make deeper knowledge more accessible to people. "I had to meet the person who devised this system. It's so deep and yet just right for beginners." What Richard Brown was also seeing and noting in those "moving leaves" was the service work the Art of Living organization does in Indian and U.S. prisons, juvenile detention centers, and rural villages, the free programs Sri Sri Ravi Shankar has created for the poorest and the most downtrodden around the world, and the fact that he has no possessions.

Richard Brown feels that the presence of a live teacher can make a difference in many people's lives, especially those who suffer from depression. But it is not necessary to have a spiritual teacher. He tells his patients who are uncomfortable with the notion of a guru to "just keep breathing," and those who follow his prescription feel better. When I finally took the Art of Living Course in Sedona with teachers Bonnie and Barry Rosen, they had a good way to explain what they were offering. They told us that we could come to the ocean with a bucket (simply learning the technique) or we could go scuba diving. In other words, the Course offers much wisdom in addition to the practice of the pranayama breathing exercises and Sudharshan Kriya. As students of the Course, we were free to accept or reject whatever served and did not serve us. We could also accept or reject Sri Sri Ravi Shankar as an "Indian man with an irritating voice," as one of the participants in my course described him, as wise teacher, as enlightened being, as the embodiment of "the love of Jesus, the silence of Buddha, the playfulness of Krishna, the wisdom of Shankara,"[11] as guru or crackpot, and however we perceived him, we could still practice the breathing.

It is my good fortune to be writing this book, because it led me to a practice from which I am deriving enormous benefit. I feel lighter than I used to, as though I'm carrying around less baggage. Yet, at the same time, there is a growing sense of strength at my core. When I attended my first advanced course at the Art of Living Canadian ashram (Art de Vivre), I met Sri Sri Ravi Shankar, a teacher of great transparency and radiance. What I mean is that there seemed to be nothing from the past weighing him down. He seemed to embrace each new moment without residue from the last one. And I'm beginning to think that the longer I practice, the more I will become like that too.

Course Philosophy

Several of Dr. Brown's severely depressed patients, whom he has referred to the Art of Living Course, not only reject the concept of a guru but are uncomfortable with the philosophical teachings as well. After taking the course, a famous scientist who has suffered from depression for most of his life told Dr. Brown that he felt much better *despite* the "Oriental philosophy" to which he had been subjected. Another patient told Dr. Brown that she couldn't stand the "Woodstock philosophy," but several months later was proposing that the Course be offered in the public schools in her community.

Others, like Suzanne, attribute their recovery from depression as much to the philosophy gleaned in the Course as to the practice of Sudharshan Kriya. Because of what she considers to be her low self-esteem, Suzanne sometimes feels she doesn't have the right to breathe, and occasionally her practice of SK becomes irregular. When this happens, her symptoms of depression return. "In the beginning, what was most dramatically helpful for me were the Course Points. If someone had just taught me these things when I was a little kid, I would have been a different person. They are such simple ideas, but they are very profound."

One of the Course Points that Suzanne finds most beneficial is "Expectation reduces the joy in life." Certainly, if you are hoping and half expecting a new bicycle or a beautiful piece of jewelry from your beloved for your birthday, you are happy when you receive it. But how much happier might you be if, on an ordinary day, not your birthday, you received such a gift? The Art of Living Course is filled with such simple observations. After taking the course, I also understood why the technique is not taught apart from the "knowledge," which includes experiential lessons in self-acceptance and compassion for self and others. The breathing experience is deepened by the philosophical components of the course, while the philosophy is understood on a deeper, more experiential level after using the breathing techniques. The Art of Living Course, like all Yogic paths, is designed to awaken us to the energy that we already are, to our connection to each other and to all beings, to living in the present moment. This awakening is accomplished not only through the technique but also through a process of exercises done with partners and in small groups, homework questions to be pondered and discussed, and through cultivating a commitment to serving others.

Taking a Daily Dose

When Suzanne doesn't practice, she feels much worse. This is not uncommon. Sometimes compliance is a problem with people suffering from severe depression, and in these cases, Richard Brown recommends that his patients repeat the course often, which Suzanne has done. One patient, who began feeling much better after practicing the breath for several months, stopped when he traveled to Germany. When he called upon his return, saying he was suicidal and asking for a change in his medication, Dr. Brown told him to resume his breathing practice. Two weeks later, when he came in for his appointment, the patient's suicidal ideas had disappeared and he was feeling good again.

Suzanne has been involved with the Art of Living for three years and feels that, as a result, she takes better care of herself, has better boundaries, and is more grounded. Despite recent major stress in her life—the effects of September 11, a breakup with her boyfriend, the suicide of a dear friend, and a new, more stressful job, "the depression is not as painful," she says, and "the anxiety seems to be gone." Her therapist and her family say they have noticed a definite change for the better in her outlook. "Usually Christmastime is unbearable for me, and this year, despite the losses in my life, my mother commented that she had never seen me so content."

When I began this chapter, I had been practicing Sudharshan Kriya every day for several weeks. Because there were no Art of Living teachers in southern Arizona at that time, I was not able to practice the hourlong Kriya, recommended in the Art of Living Course. Still, I noticed that I felt more energy and yet was more relaxed about writing this book, able to pace my work on this and other projects without the mild anxiety I sometimes feel when faced with deadlines. I wrote a draft of this chapter after my return from my first Advanced Course at the Canadian ashram in Quebec, where Sri Sri Ravi Shankar led meditations and group processes, and spoke regularly about the love that is available to us all, all the time. Now I have been practicing SK every day, along with my asana, pranayama, and meditation practice, for eight months. I hardly recognize myself as the Amy who believed she would always have "empty pockets." As I write this I am deeply saddened by events in my personal life and in our country. But my grief is like the changing weather. What I know is that the fullness I feel in my abiding connection to Self with a capital *S* comes from the deep wellspring of love of which Sri Sri speaks. My abundance is real. The suffering I felt was impermanent as the clouds over my head. And here in Tucson, the sky is mostly clear.

One cautionary note: It is known that lithium is excreted during mechanical hyperventilation, making it less available to the brain. Although Sudharshan Kriya is not a hyperventilation technique, a portion of the practice may have a similar effect on lithium secretion. Therefore, if you are suffering from bipolar disorder and are prone to manic episodes, consult with a psychiatrist before learning SK. With your doctor's help, you may be able to adjust the level of your medication to accommodate the practice. All other aspects of the course—the pranayama, the philosophical teachings, and the chanting—can be beneficial and most likely do not affect lithium levels.

yoga experience

I am not an Art of Living teacher, so I cannot teach you here or in person how to practice Sudharshan Kriya, the variation of ujjayi called Three-Stage Breathing, or the version of Bhastrika taught in their program. To learn these techniques, you must take the Art of Living Course.

Pulling Prana

"Pulling Prana" shares some similarities with Bhastrika and likely has a similar effect. It is an energizing breathing technique I learned as a guest at Kripalu in the late eighties and one that my students enjoy. The vagus nerve is likely stimulated, and there is a probable release of the "feel-good" hormones oxytocin and prolactin.

Stand with your feet a comfortable distance apart. Inhale deeply through your nostrils while extending your arms straight out in front of you with your fingers spread wide and your palms facing up. Make fists of your hands and vigorously draw them back to your waist with a forceful exhalation through your nostrils. Do this twenty times, then let your arms float to your sides. Close your eyes and bathe in the effects of prana flooding your cells.

You can repeat the sequence, practicing no more than three rounds. You can also vary the exercise by pulling the prana from above your head. You may also alternate right and left arms. Always, when you complete a round, take time to close your eyes and absorb the effects.

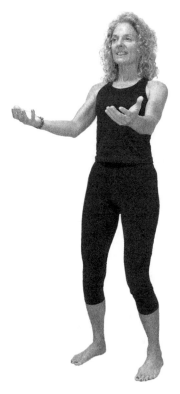 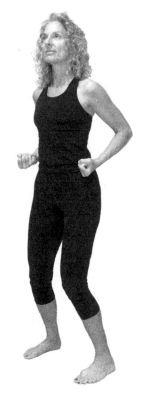

Pulling Prana: Inhale arms up   *Pulling Prana: Exhale vigorously*

meditate to mediate

When milk is poured into milk, oil into oil, water into water,
they blend in absolute oneness. So also . . . the spiritual seeker
who meditates on the *Atman* becomes the Atman.

—*Shankara's Crest-Jewel of Discrimination*[1]

The rest-note,
unwritten,
hinged between worlds,
that precedes change and allows it.

—JANE HIRSHFIELD, from "The Door," *The October Palace*[2]

Ecstasy as a State of Mind

When we discussed the Eight-Limbed Path outlined in Patanjali's
Yoga Sutras in Chapter Four, we looked most closely at the first
four limbs of yoga—yama (restraint), niyama (observance), asana (posture), and pranayama (breath control). In this chapter we'll explore the
final four limbs, which create a calm, healing state in body and mind,
containing and even ameliorating depression and anxiety. The final
four limbs are *pratyahara* (withdrawal of the senses), *dharana* (concentration), *dhyana* (meditation), and *samadhyaya* (total absorption or superconscious states). As we've seen, the first four limbs help release tension

and trauma stored in our bodies. In practicing the final four limbs, we continue to balance and purify the mind.

Pratyahara, or withdrawal of the senses, may be achieved in the practice of the asana. You don't have to sit on a meditation cushion to experience the effects of closing your eyes and allowing your mind to be absorbed in the sensations you're feeling in a pose. For some people, especially those suffering from major depression or PTSD, techniques that cultivate pratyahara and dharana (concentration) may be the most efficient means of returning to a calm and focused state of mind. Meditation, or dhyana, may be too difficult when the mind is caught in the obsessive turmoil of depressive thoughts.

The final limb that Patanjali discusses is *samadhyaya*, or surrender into the state of wholeness. This is not a state reserved for the meditation cushion either. Perhaps you've felt this oneness while observing a butterfly landing on a fragrant bloom, while slicing a mango, or while following the flight of a bird. Perhaps you've felt this wholeness as you gazed into the eyes of a baby or a lover or a spiritual teacher. Once, while sitting on a hill near Vivekanandra Kendra, the Yoga treatment and research center outside Mysore, I watched a hawk in flight. But "watched" doesn't describe the flight I felt in the muscles of my shoulders, the wave of breath within me and without, bearing me aloft. Of course, I hadn't moved from my place on the rock, but my spirit was in union with that bird.

This state of grace is our birthright, not just some spiritual high. The practices we do simply strip away the obstacles we've accumulated in our daily lives, so that we can be conscious of our wholeness even in our disappointments and our pain. As I suggested in Chapter Four, I don't believe the eight limbs described by Patanjali are rungs of a ladder leading to a final goal of wholeness. Rather, they are to be practiced simultaneously, the way a tree grows its branches. We have access to the eighth limb, *samadhi*, whether we are practicing Yoga or meditating or not. We can experience that sense of oneness in any activity, in every activity, even in our sorrow, on the Yoga mat and off. But the practices of Yoga, including meditation, will purify your mind and body so that there is less constriction, less room for depression, and more room to experience the ecstasy of your wholeness, to experience your own *samadhi* in every moment of your life. Meditation teachers from most traditions have a similar attitude toward this state of mind (or no-mind in the Buddhist tradition). John Tarrant, who is a Zen Roshi, an author, and was a depth psychologist for many years, puts it this way: "That state is something that is happening and available all the time. We merely notice it more when we use special methods. It gives us a taste of what it's like not to be in conflict inside, to be open to what's happening. We feel more energy, we are more creative and the mind is clearer."

Whether you have an anxiety-based depression, have bipolar disorder, or suffer from dysthymia, major depression, or PTSD, there are meditation techniques that can help you balance your mood. You may not cure the depression with your practice, but meditation can be a form of mediating with those negative mind states, negotiating with your depression so it doesn't control your life. For the most part, the more calming forms of meditation, which we'll look at first, benefit everyone. There is a large body of research that for more than thirty years has documented the effectiveness of the calming mantra-based meditation techniques like Transcendental Meditation and the Relaxation Response in treating hypertension, heart disease, and anxiety. For more than twenty years, hundreds of studies based on Jon Kabat-Zinn's Stress Reduction and Relaxation Program (SRRP), conducted by the Mindfulness-Based Stress Reduction Clinic at the University of Massachusetts Medical School in Worcester and by research institutions throughout the world, have shown that mindfulness meditation is equally effective in treating these ailments. But if you are suffering from major depression or PTSD, you might be better off learning one of the more active techniques we'll discuss later in the chapter.

Mindfulness

Mindfulness practice is a way of observing and slowly quieting the active monkey mind. The ancient texts compare the activity of the mind to a monkey that has been stung by a scorpion. We leap from thought to thought, or worry a thought until it wrings us out. When we sit to practice mindfulness meditation, we give the monkey a chance to slow down. Usually, mindfulness is first taught with attention to the breath. You attend to the sensation of breath moving in and out at the tip of your nostrils, or, if it is easier, you may observe the way the belly moves with the breath. Your mind will wander. That's what the mind does. But when you notice that you are thinking again, you invite your attention back to the breath. Eventually, when the mind is calmed by attention to the breath, you may practice mindfulness by attending to the passing thoughts, the sensations in your body, the rise and fall of feelings. Mindfulness teachers call this "Choiceless Awareness." In this practice, you can learn a lot about your various mind states, and, as such, it is a form of self-study (svadhyaya), or insight.

Mindfulness is the technique used in Insight Meditation (Vipassana in Pali), and is said to be the technique practiced by the Buddha. The theory behind Insight Meditation is that when we practice mindfulness, we begin to develop insight into the nature of the self and the universe. The simplest example given is that if you have never meditated before and close your eyes and are quiet, the first insight that may come is that the mind jumps all over the place and is less in your control than you might have imagined. As you watch your thoughts and feelings rise and fall, the idea of impermanence is revealed.

Vipassana Meditation teacher, author, and psychotherapist Sylvia Boorstein told me about a friend and fellow psychotherapist, a woman who had a lifelong cyclical depression—very likely genetic, inherited from her mother—who, through the help of her mindfulness practice, was able to manage her life skillfully. She would recognize an oncoming bout of depression and organize her life so that she could accommodate it. In recent years, the availability of appropriate drugs for her depression has alleviated most of her symptoms. Sylvia's friend reports that she is now able to use her meditation practice "to see profoundly into the nature of things as they really are, because I don't have to use up so much energy just holding myself together." "I believe that mindfulness helped," Sylvia says, "in the years before drugs were available, because she could stop fighting with her depression. Or being mad at herself for being depressed."

When, over time, we observe our thoughts, it is easy to see that much of our reactions to our present circumstances are the result of the stories we have made out of the events of our lives. We have stories about our childhoods that rationalize our adult behavior. We have stories about our relationships that explain their failures to ourselves. What would happen if we dropped our stories? Might we be able to engage with others without the limits of our preconceived notions about the way things usually turn out? A sitting practice can help us do that. In Yogic terms, this is the self-study (*svadhyaya*) we discussed in Chapter Four, that self-awareness so essential in removing the obstacles to our freedom. We can begin to understand a little more about our patterns of behavior and states of mind when we are able to observe the mind in meditation practice.

Mindfulness for Anxiety-Based Depression

Rachel, a thirty-six-year-old law librarian, grew up in a chaotic household. Her mother was an alcoholic who would not confront her dermatologist husband about his nightly erotic massages of Rachel. To the Jewish community, Rachel's family appeared intact and loving. After all, until Sue Silverman blew the lid off dysfunctional Jewish families in her best-selling memoir, *Because I Remember Terror, Father, I Remember You*, there was "no such thing" as alcoholism or incest among Jews. As Rachel was growing up, she developed an irrational fear of the dark, likely a projection outward of how unsafe it felt to live in her body. For years, into adulthood, she could not go into a dark room alone. Sitting in a movie theater when the lights went down was momentarily terrifying. In addition to her fears, she had a great deal of trouble making decisions. Though an excellent student, she floated from college to college, graduate program to graduate program, until she finally earned a master's degree in library science—a field that she says helped her organize her chaotic universe. "It took me a long time to earn a degree. I was always afraid I would choose the wrong course, and the rest of my life would be ruined. If I chose course A, then I couldn't take course B, which felt limiting. Every time I had to make a decision—an apartment, a course, whether to take a part-time job or a student loan—the uncertainty drove me crazy. I became irritable, anxious, and depressed."

In his book *Going to Pieces Without Falling Apart*, Mark Epstein cites the work of psychoanalyst D. W. Winnicott. "Winnicott taught that to go willingly into unknowing was the key to living a full life."[3] Rachel could not go into unknowing without terror, because she had not developed what Winnicott called "good-enough ego coverage." "Only if a parent provides 'good-enough ego coverage' can a child go without fear into the unknown."[4] Rachel could not even tolerate her own feelings, fearing that they would overwhelm her. She controlled her emotions by organizing all the externals that she could—books, food, activities with her friends. She stayed active, leading a busy social life where she rarely had to be alone. "To bless the imperfect, to enter the not-knowing, is to make a voluntary return to darkness, the source," says John Tarrant.[5] But Rachel was afraid of the dark.

After taking six years to complete her undergraduate degree, then experiencing extreme anxiety about her future when she did so, Rachel went to work on herself. She began to see a therapist who practiced mindfulness meditation. After six months of therapy and three months of mindfulness practice, she went to her first ten-day meditation course at an isolated retreat center in rural New England. Rachel found sitting still on a cushion with her eyes closed extremely uncomfortable. When she talked with her meditation teacher about her discomfort, he encouraged her to sit, observing the breath with her eyes open. "If I hadn't trusted my therapist and wanted his approval, I probably would have bolted after a day of sitting with my eyes closed. But practicing mindfulness with my eyes open made me feel safe and eventually created a calm inner state. By the end of the retreat, I was sitting with my eyes closed."

"Mindfulness meditation does not require closing one's eyes, although often people find that comfortable," says Sylvia Boorstein. "I usually close my eyes when I am sitting, but I open them if I am sleepy. I can still be paying attention to my process; I can feel my body; I can feel my breath; I can attend to my mind states." Though most people refer to meditation as "sitting," one can practice mindfulness in any position. "A person could think of themselves as a mindfulness practitioner," says Sylvia, "and never sit down. You could walk for your entire practice. You can cook mindfully, clean house mindfully, do any job mindfully. Mindfulness is the practice of paying attention with the hope of seeing more clearly what is happening inside and outside. If I see more clearly, I will be able to respond in a way that doesn't cause suffering to myself or anyone else."

When Buddhist psychiatrist and author Mark Epstein was a beginning meditator, anxious about making the grade as a sophomore at Harvard, he learned to "use awareness of my breathing as a model for attention to difficult emotional states."[6] A practice that observes without judgment the thoughts and feelings that arise in the mind allows the meditator to begin to witness the fluctuating states of mind without reacting to them. For Rachel, learning to meditate was a tremendous relief. She began to attend to her conflicted thoughts, her indecision, even her fear of the unknown, with less anxiety. As her meditation practice developed, Rachel became increasingly able to tolerate change and uncertainty in her life. "To this day, I have trouble making decisions, but I can laugh about it. I don't fall apart the way I did ten years ago."

After several years of practice, deep and troubling images from her childhood sexual abuse began to surface when Rachel went on retreat. With the help of her therapist and her meditation teacher, who again suggested that she practice with her eyes open, she was able to face her childhood trauma without succumbing to the anxiety and depression it originally produced. Rachel doesn't experience less grief in her life since she began her practice. In fact, she says she is more aware of grief and anger than she was when she struggled to avoid it. "I understand now that my feelings are an appropriate response to my childhood and to the sometimes difficult circumstances I face today, and I don't have to hang on to them. If I can go deeper into my grief on my meditation cushion, I can move through it. I don't have to fear that I will never stop crying." With the help of a therapist, Rachel was strong enough to sit with her pain.

Pain doesn't go away as a result of a meditation practice. Even long-term meditators experience the ordinary losses that being human entails. However, the recognition of impermanence that comes with meditation practice helps support the understanding that the pain will pass. We don't need to identify with our pain, our depression, or even our negative thoughts about ourselves. We don't have to suffer more *because* we're in pain, which is what happens when we find ourselves unable to acknowledge and simply accept the pain. Sitting in meditation, attending to the passing thoughts and feelings, helps us notice just how fleeting our feeling states are. "I'm not hoping for the end of pain," says Sylvia. "That does not happen in anyone's life. I'm working on establishing a good relationship with pain. The central teaching of the Buddha is that there *is* pain. Suffering is resistance to the pain; suffering is struggling with the pain; suffering is saying that it should be otherwise. Don't talk about the end of pain. Talk about the end of the struggle with what is."

Mindfulness for Dysthymia

The only thing that is permanent, Yogi Amrit Desai used to say, is impermanence. Everything changes. When we cling to what we have, we create suffering for ourselves. When we yearn for what we cannot have, we create suffering for ourselves. But when we can begin to accept that nothing we have—relationships, looks, possessions—is permanent, that we live in a world of change, we can begin to accept life as it is. Edward is a retired lawyer in Rhode Island with a history of dysthymic depression and cyclical bouts of major depression who is learning this lesson through his Vipassana meditation practice. The early loss of his parents—his mother died of cancer when he was four and his father died of a heart attack when Edward was eleven—created within him a sense of loneliness and a fear of abandonment he has carried for most of his life. For many years, Edward unconsciously guarded himself against deeply engaging with anyone who might disappoint him, fending off abandonment by remaining alone. He had friends and lovers, and a brief marriage in his twenties, but even in that relationship he maintained some distance, unconsciously holding back lest his companion betray him.

When he retired early from his law practice seven years ago, he began a Vipassana meditation practice, and more recently, he began practicing Yoga. As he began to sit in meditation, observing his breath, attending to the sensations in his body and the thoughts passing through his mind, his knowledge of the changing, impermanent nature of his own thoughts and feelings grew. With that dawning knowledge, his expectation for permanence gradually diminished along with some of his fear, and he was able to engage more deeply, forming relationships that he believes are less constricted by his fear of loss.

During a trip to Europe, he let his practice lapse and, when we spoke, had not been meditating regularly for several weeks. "I am very clear what difference it makes when I do practice." When he practices daily, sitting in the morning for sometimes as long as forty minutes, he says it sets a tone for the day. He's relatively calm throughout the day and able to cultivate an attitude of "being okay with whatever is happening." Even when he feels uncomfortable—"feeling lonely, feeling bored, feeling upset about something"—if he acknowledges his discomfort, if he doesn't resist what is happening, the discomfort usually fades.

"When I'm able to observe whatever is happening and let it be okay, life is a lot easier. I get a lot less tense and a lot less depressed. Things don't stick and my life goes more smoothly."

As we talked, he reflected on how much tension had built up in the weeks that he hadn't practiced, and how much more anxiety he had been feeling as a result. "All sorts of little fears come up during the course of the day, which, if I'm practicing and paying attention, I can say, 'Oh, that's fear,' and let it go. If I'm not practicing, then it builds and I start closing down. I feel driven by whatever is going on in my mind; there's more tightness in my body, and I lose my sense of expansion." This becomes a spiral downward for Edward. When he goes too long without practicing, he feels contracted, physically and emotionally, and it becomes more difficult to sit in meditation. "When I'm depressed, there's much more resistance to sitting, much more resistance to watching my mind." That's when he turns to Hatha Yoga.

When he can bring himself to Yoga class, even if he is feeling depressed, there's a sense that something different is possible. "I begin to actually feel the energy in my body. Being in touch with what's going on in my body through Yoga postures teaches me what's going on with my depression." When Edward returned from his trip to Europe, he was feeling depressed and unable to sit in meditation. Resuming his Yoga practice gave him the opportunity to locate the heaviness in his body that accompanied the depression. "Once I started stretching and breathing more deeply, I began to feel a sense of expansion, which gave me a concrete experience of how contracted I had become."

When he begins with the physical, which for Edward includes vigorous and lung-expanding pranayama breathing like Prana Pulling and Skull-Shining Breath (kapalabhati) and heart-opening backbends, he finds it easier to resume his sitting practice and to once again begin to acknowledge and accept whatever is happening throughout the rest of his day—in all its glorious impermanence.

Though, unlike Edward, most of us have grown up with parents, many of us are familiar with the feeling of closing down rather than taking the risk of connecting deeply with another human being. We want to push away what is painful, but when we close off to our pain, protecting ourselves from suffering, we reduce our capacity for joy as well as our ability to connect with others. A sitting meditation practice that cultivates self-observation allows us to pay attention to *all* our feelings. When we do so, we begin to feel more real. When the heart is closed, we live unaffected by the beauty of a sunset or the blooming of an orchid. We are numb to the multitude of offerings from the natural world. And we begin to feel unreal to ourselves. Cultivating a practice that lets us feel calmer allows us to stay present to our feelings, so that we can take in and really feel the sense of joy at simple pleasures—the sight of a lone cow on a hill at sunset, the voice of an old friend on the phone, the smell of orange blossoms on a bike ride through the neighborhood. This is what it means to be alive.

Zen Meditation

Screenwriter and college teacher Annina Lavee has struggled with feelings of depression for most of her life, compounded when she lost her husband to lung cancer twenty-four years ago. She has been practicing Zen meditation for six years. "My form of depression," she says, "is getting caught up in an obsessive cycle of whatever the issue is for me at that particular time." When she meditates on the breath or a *koan*, which is a question or riddle that has no rational answer, usually posed by the Zen master, it interrupts her obsessive thought pattern and broadens her perspective. "My practice opens up the blinders that depression creates for me." During the grief incurred by a recent breakup of a long-term relationship, Annina found herself sitting to meditate with a koan often, sometimes three times a day, to help her break through the troubling repetition of thoughts about the relationship.

Her teacher, John Tarrant, suggests that meditators who experience the kind of obsessive thinking that Annina describes work with their thoughts on and off the cushion. "I do like people to do sitting meditation every day, but the practice of being a person walking the journey of transformation is something that goes on all the time. It's about being more alive; it's not about sitting down and breathing a certain way. If the obsessive thoughts are making you less alive, then it doesn't matter where they're occurring. You work with them, challenging them, wherever and whenever they arise." On the cushion, he suggests several techniques for working with recurring thoughts. First, he says that it doesn't hurt for the meditator to notice what she's thinking—"Now I'm thinking happy thoughts," or "now I'm remembering something," for example. The usefulness in labeling your thoughts in this way is that you begin to notice how transitory they are. Second, he suggests that just sitting, "not opposing your thoughts, but not paying a lot of attention to them, either," can allow them to shift.

The method he prefers and uses in his teaching is the practice of *koans*. "With a koan, you engage with it under any condition. It really doesn't matter if you're happy or you're sad or you've got cancer or you're bored or you're getting married. Life is there and the koan just goes with the quirkiness of life, the strangeness of life and allows us to find the richness in any circumstance." One koan that Tarrant uses is the word *no*. Any ruminative thought that arises, causing you discomfort or sorrow or pain, "you notice the thought," he says, "then you bring it up against 'no.'" The idea behind this koan is to challenge the thought that is causing you unhappiness. When you do this, Tarrant says, "you'll find that the thought usually isn't entirely true. Happiness takes care of itself, if you challenge the belief system."

The ancient Buddhist teachings upon which Tarrant's teaching of Zen are founded sound a bit like cognitive therapy here. Yet, he says, there's an aspect of the use of koans that isn't present in most psychotherapy, including cognitive therapy, in which you directly confront your negative thoughts and limiting beliefs. "Koans harmonize with the weirdness of the world. Cognitive therapy is very rational, but the world isn't rational. Intuitively, we know that. That's why we have poetry and music. Koans are more like that. If you stay with the koan, if you let it in, then it becomes metaphor; it goes beyond 'yes' and 'no.' Mental health is always a normative kind of thing and tends to cut out the poetry and genius that everybody has. The nice thing about koans is that they allow people's genius to come out. Koans allow for the unexpected, actually embrace it."

Unlike some other teachers who warn against a sitting practice for PTSD, Tarrant feels that using a koan form of meditation can actually be beneficial. He feels that flashbacks are not a problem in and of themselves. "They're just images. Assuming you're not psychotic, Zen meditation can be great. It stops you stressing out. It stops you identifying with every thought, feeling, and image that comes through. Koan meditation, in particular, can help you question the thoughts associated with the traumatic experience. Through koan meditation you can begin to question your habit of bringing your past suffering into your everyday experience when the causes of that suffering aren't here anymore."

Mantra Transmission

Some meditation techniques use a word or phrase or sound, which is called a *mantra,* as the focus point for the mind. Sometimes the mantra is arbitrarily picked by the meditator, or the mantra can be given by a meditation teacher. In some traditions, the transmission of the mantra becomes a ritual, and is passed in secrecy from teacher to student. Jim Larsen is grounded in a mantra-based meditation tradition. He has practiced Transcendental Meditation (TM) daily since 1973, when he received his mantra in secret from a teacher trained by Maharishi Mahesh Yogi, who brought this mantra-based system of meditation to the West in the late sixties. Jim taught Transcendental Meditation for seventeen years, and then in 1993 was initiated by his guru, Sri Sri Ravi Shankar, in the meditation practice of *Sahaj Samadhi,* a heart-centered form of mantra meditation taught by the Art of Living Foundation. Both TM and Sahaj Samadhi are based on the principle of effortlessly witnessing the mind with periodic introduction of a mantra. Since 1993 he has taught Sahaj Samadhi and feels there is a significant difference between a technique in which you choose your own mantra or are given one arbitrarily and the transmission that takes place when you receive a mantra from an enlightened spiritual master. "Initiating a relaxation response in the mind," he says, "can be achieved in many ways because it is natural for the mind to relax. But when meditation is practiced with a mantra received from an enlightened master, or a teacher authorized to pass on the mantra from the master, the practice has another component. The master infuses the mantra with his *shakti* [energy or consciousness]."

There's no evidence that your symptoms will improve faster or more completely if you are given a mantra by a revered teacher or if you pick one from your favorite song, but there is the issue of faith, and faith alone can be a potent healer. There is a body of research that suggests that religious faith, whatever its content, can support someone through an illness, and that people with faith have a higher rate of recovery from serious illness than people without religious belief. So if you believe that your mantra is infused with the energy of your beloved teacher, then your recovery may be hastened by that faith.

But I do believe that there are some people on the planet who have, through their energy, the power to heal others. There is nothing scientific in my belief, of course, yet I have seen people release their suffering in the presence of a beloved teacher. It could be argued that the healing "miracles" that occur in the presence of certain beings are the result of faith and not the energy inherent in the Guru or healer. On the other hand, I hold out the possibility that such "miracles" may in part be the result of the energy—call it Shakti, call it divine, call it love—flowing through the healer.

Mantra-based meditation was the first practice I learned. In 1969, when I was a freshman in college, I had trouble sleeping. In part, my insomnia may have been the result of the stress of being a student away from home for the first time in an era of political protest and free love. Certainly, the values I had carried with me from my suburban childhood and adolescence were in conflict with the prevailing mores. For my second semester, I transferred to another school, further disrupting my equilibrium and adding to my stress. But I was fortunate to begin dating a fellow student who complemented his pot smoking with Transcendental Meditation. Since my first experience with pot led me to believe my arm was falling off, I chose to enhance our togetherness by learning to meditate. I was given my own personal mantra by my meditation teacher and was told to allow my mind to hold that single syllable for twenty minutes twice a day. Of course, my mind wandered, but when I remembered, I brought my attention back to my mantra. Within weeks, I found I was sleeping better. There is good reason for this. Unlike people who are mentally healthy, people who are depressed have increased rapid eye movement (REM) early in the sleep period, and it takes people suffering from mania longer for (REM) to begin.[7] Meditation has also been shown to help restore normal sleep patterns. In a recent study conducted by the University of California at San Diego that looked at the management of sleep abnormalities during periods of abstinence in alcohol-dependent patients, meditation was recommended as a way to normalize sleep patterns.[8]

Healing State

Let's set aside the talk about the differences in meditation techniques and talk about the commonalities. Sometimes, during practice, the active mind slips away from its moorings and we seem to float for several moments in a state of ease, often not recognizing we've been there until the anchor of conscious thought pulls the mind to the surface once again. We notice we are thinking and recognize that for a timeless moment our minds were suspended. This is the relaxed state of increased alpha waves in the brain, measured in practitioners of Transcendental Meditation. The overvigilant thinking mind relaxes and we are in a state of grace. This is the state that will heal us.

With the regular practice of calming meditation techniques like Transcendental Meditation, Sahaj Samadhi, Vipassana or mindfulness meditation, Zen meditation, and the numerous meditation techniques taught as Jewish meditation, Christian meditation, and Native American Meditation, among others, we have access to this state. The subjective experience is a floaty feeling in the mind, similar to a runner's high or the relaxed state experienced just after orgasm. This is a healthy state where mind and body are aligned. This is the healing state that the ancient Yogis called *samadhi*. Despite the troubles of daily life, when you sit, paying attention to your breath, or attuning to a mantra, or observing the sensations in your body or the thoughts in your mind, you have the opportunity to touch, for a moment, that deep abiding state of wholeness at your core. Coming home to this feeling every day can create a calm center, a peaceful container for the passing difficulties in your life.

Too often, we fear that if we let ourselves dive into such a deep state of consciousness, we will never emerge. We will lose our identity or our grasp on reality. But as we struggle to stay in control, we feel more and more separate from reality. It is in this ability to lose ourselves that we find the fullness of who we are. Practicing this dissolving of self on the meditation cushion enhances our capacity to let go, to be more creative, to dance and sing without self-consciousness, to fully relax and enjoy our sexual experiences. Mark Epstein says that it is "one of the most important tasks of adulthood to discover, or rediscover, the ability to lose oneself."[9] He goes on to say that when we are afraid to relax the mind's vigilance, "we tend to equate this floating with drowning and we start to founder. In this fear, we destroy our capacity to discover ourselves in a new way. We doom ourselves to a perpetual hardening of character, which we imagine is sanity, but which comes to imprison us."[10]

"The conventional wisdom about mindfulness," says Sylvia Boorstein, "is that you become liberated from your old mind habits as you see clearly how those habits work to create suffering. Seeing clearly—insight—is what mattered most. That's what I've been teaching for years, but more recently I've come to believe that it's a combination of seeing clearly and absorption in resting mind states. Afflictive emotions seem to be soothed, to become less potent, when the mind 'rests' for periods of time in *samadhi*, deep concentration." There is now medical evidence to support what Sylvia has come, over the twenty years that she's been teaching meditation, to believe.

Whether the attention is maintained internally, as on thoughts or the breath or on a mantra, or externally on an object, all forms of contemplative Yoga share a method of one-pointed awareness (*dharana*). When the attention is one-pointed, the mind is calmed and anxiety is reduced. "Meditation," says Stanford psychiatrist Roy King and his colleague Ann Brownstone, "can inhibit ongoing and distracting thoughts, feelings and images. This inhibitory process can ameliorate the negative effect and negative cognitions that plague those suffering from chronic stress conditions and anxiety disorders."[11]

Research done by Dr. Richard Davidson, director of the Laboratory for Affective Neuroscience at the University of Wisconsin, demonstrates that the location of brain activity determines our moods, and that mindfulness meditation has the potential to change the location of our brain activity. Using functional MRI and advanced EEG analysis, Dr. Davidson has determined that when people are emotionally distressed, suffering from either anxiety or depression or both, they have more activity in the amygdala, at the center of the limbic or emotional brain, and the right prefrontal cortex. By contrast, happy people have more activity in the left prefrontal cortex. According to psychologist and author Daniel Goleman, Dr. Davidson has shown "a quick way to index a person's typical mood range, by reading the baseline levels of activity in these right and left prefrontal areas. That ratio predicts daily moods with surprising accuracy. The more the ratio tilts to the right, the more unhappy or distressed a person tends to be, while the more activity to the left, the more happy and enthusiastic."[12]

The most exciting news comes from a recent controlled study that Dr. Davidson did in collaboration with Jon Kabat-Zinn, in which mindfulness meditation was taught to workers in a high-pressure biotech business for roughly three hours a week over two months. Before the mindfulness training, the workers showed high levels of emotional stress and their brain scans showed more activity in the right prefrontal cortex. After the training in mindfulness, on average their brain scans showed more activity on the left side. "Simultaneously, their moods improved; they reported feeling engaged again in their work, more energized and less anxious."[13] What this study shows is that with proper training, mindfulness meditation can shift the biological set of our brains, so that our brains, regardless of the circumstances of our lives, are programmed to be less anxious and depressed and more positive and upbeat.

Hamburger Thoughts

But lest you think that meditation is always about dissolving on your cushion or that it feels easy while you're practicing, let me tell you about my own early Vipassana experiences, when my mind seemed bound to my body's discomfort. At my first meditation retreat at Kripalu in the late eighties, we were practicing a mindfulness form of meditation. Though I was an irregular practitioner of TM, I had never simply paid attention to the breath, never sat observing the sensations in my body. I went to the retreat after a mild illness, and sitting was difficult. It was hard to merely witness the discomfort. I sat on a cushion, observing the pain in my right knee until tears were rolling down my face. I wasn't witnessing. I was in it! After that morning session, I went for a long walk in the woods around Kripalu Center. This was not specifically a walking meditation as practiced on many Vipassana and Zen retreats. I was simply getting some exercise on a mild spring day, albeit slowly. I began to see the radiance of the filtered light upon the leaves, smell the mossy loam beneath my feet, hear an animal rooting in the undergrowth, and it was all so wonderful. I felt alive and deeply, intimately connected to everything around me. I was the bark of the pine tree, the fallen acorn, the returning robin. There was no separation. What I realized was that though the actual meditation experience had been gruesome, something had been released in me as I sat in discomfort on my cushion, so that I felt more fully myself and could see that Self in all things.

No matter what form of meditation you may practice, there are days when the mind is spinning—hamburger thoughts, I used to call them when I led noon meditation sessions at Kripalu. But just noticing the spin, perhaps labeling it—"thinking," "fear," "fantasy"—can slow the rpm of your thoughts. Even if there are no momentary dips into samadhi-land, after meditating for twenty minutes or so, the mind will be clearer, calmer.

Retreat

After you have been meditating regularly for several months, you might find that attending a meditation retreat can boost your enthusiasm for your practice and deepen your experience on the meditation cushion. A meditation retreat, according to John Tarrant, "puts a container around your experience so that you can go deep." You don't have to answer your cell phone or your e-mails. "A retreat can allow us to live from what we can't conceive of, rather than what we can. New possibilities can occur and we become more creative. The new line of the poem or the bar of music comes from out of the unknown, from what is not conceivable."

I experienced a way to live from a heretofore-unknown possibility, something that before my retreat remained inconceivable to me. I was on a nine-day personal retreat in a tiny meditation cabin in the mountains above Boulder, Colorado. A personal retreat differs from an ordinary meditation retreat in that you really are alone. This is not recommended for someone new to meditation practice, or even for an experienced meditator who has not had experience in group meditation retreats. It is especially not recommended for someone in the throes of depression or who suffers from PTSD. When you are depressed, spending so much time alone can feel tremendously isolating. But I had already spent a week in a semisilent meditation retreat with Rabbi David and Shoshana Cooper in Fort Collins, Colorado, during a large Jewish Renewal conference, so I followed them back to their home in the Rockies where they facilitate personal retreats for experienced individual practitioners. David is the author of many books about meditation, *Kabbalah,* and the spiritual journey, including *A Heart of Stillness* and *God Is a Verb.* Together the Coopers teach meditation retreats in the Jewish mystical tradition. The rugged, forested terrain, lush with aspen and pine trees, was so spectacular that I expected to intersperse my time in sitting meditation with walks through the woods. I took exactly one walk on the day of my arrival. After that, I used the time to go deeper inside, to sit with my breath, alternating rounds of meditation with Yoga and occasionally writing in my journal. I spoke only for about ten minutes every other day, when I met briefly with David or Shoshana in their home. Contrary to my expectations, I had no particular insights that applied to my own pressing issues. I spent the time feeling so much bigger than the petty concerns with which I'd arrived. I spent the time in a healing place, an unexpectedly peaceful place. After the retreat, the questions I had carried to Colorado seemed to resolve themselves with little effort. It became clear to me that I would find tenants for my house in Rhode Island and move to the Southwest, where the expansive sky mirrored my state of mind.

Not all meditation retreats are so peaceful or produce such major transitions. I spent one five-day Vipassana retreat with teacher Eric Kolvig, immersed in grief, as I began to realize that my four-year relationship was never going to meet my needs and that the house my partner and I had purchased together would have to be sold. Eric cautioned me against making major decisions while on retreat, but my resolve held over the weeks after my return, and a month later, my partner and I began a yearlong process of separating.

Edward, the retired lawyer in Rhode Island, goes on five- to ten-day Vipassana retreats several times a year and last year spent thirty days on a meditation retreat at Spirit Rock in California. His experience on retreat has been as varied as the events of his life. There have been moments of breakthrough, moments of joy, as well as moments spent in grief and in anger. But what is consistent throughout is his awareness of the impermanence of his feelings. "One of the most valuable aspects of the practice is that it allows me to have feelings, which in the past I would have blocked. I can see, when I meditate, when I am blocking something, and that can allow me to open to the feeling, to allow it to flow and complete itself. My practice allows me to not be so identified with a feeling that I get lost in it."

This ability to not identify with his feelings stood him in good stead when he was on the thirty-day retreat. Throughout the month of silence, he would often see a man walking with a hangdog expression on his face. The sight of the man would annoy Edward to the point of what seemed to him a totally out-of-proportion response. What he began to realize was that the man's victimlike demeanor was triggering his rage at his own tendency to see himself as the victim of his life story. This was confirmed for Edward after the retreat when he made it a point to meet and talk to the man. In fact, the man was quite assertive in his life, not a victim at all. During the retreat, Edward had projected his own unresolved feelings onto the man, a process that allowed him to confront his own lack of acceptance for his legitimate grief over his losses.

On a recent retreat with Vipassana meditation teacher Phillip Moffitt, Edward became aware, as he sat with the chronic pain in his jaw, that the tension he had been carrying in his body since childhood was there for a reason. "I began to see that this pain had actually been an ally for me. I recognized that the need to stuff a lot of my feelings when I was a child was essential for my survival." When he spoke with Phillip about it, Phillip agreed. He suggested to Edward that the pain and tension were a repository of the feelings that were not safe to express in the hostile environment in which, after his parents died, he was raised. Phillip advised him to be gentle with the tension. "For years, I had been refusing to accept this pain, trying to get rid of it in many different ways. A shift occurred when I recognized that the pain had been almost a lifesaver for me at the time. What emerged out of that was an incredible tenderness for myself as a young child." Since the retreat, Edward has been able to reconcile himself to the tension in his jaw and it has actually lessened.

It's often not a good idea to go on a meditation retreat when you are in the midst of grieving a loss or in a major depressive episode. When someone is grieving, she needs people around her. He needs comforting talk and soothing touch. Vipassana retreats are held in silence, with no social contact between retreatants. "A Vipassana retreat can be extremely hard," says Sylvia Boorstein. "When someone you love has just died, there's a grief and mourning period that is appropriately done with other people. Someone in grief needs holding, needs not to be alone, and a certain amount of moving around." The objectives of a meditation retreat—being alone with your own mind, silence, stillness—are very different from the needs of someone who is mourning.

But when the initial stages of grief have been completed, going on a retreat may be soothing, offering a respite to continually being obligated to speak of the loss. Responses to retreat circumstances are idiosyncratic. "It's hard to determine for anyone what their response will be," says Sylvia, "especially if they are recuperating from a loss. Either it's a little bit soothing because silence is soothing and the dharma [the wisdom of the teachings derived from the Buddha] is so consoling to listen to. Or it's depressing because everybody else looks exhalted, and you feel as though you're in the worst mind-state in the world." Some meditation teachers, whether they are also psychotherapists like Sylvia or not, are comfortable supporting people through such conflicted states of mind during retreat. Others are less comfortable.

If you are in a state of depression, it is best to talk with the meditation teacher beforehand to determine if the retreat will be appropriate for you. And just as it's important to find a qualified Yoga teacher who supports and encourages your healing, it's equally important to find a kind and patient meditation teacher, willing to work with you if you suffer from depression. "There are meditation teachers I know," says Sylvia, "who are tremendously skilled and tremendously interested and patient in working with emerging trauma, and see it as part of the healing of the whole being. On the other hand, there are more classically oriented people who will say, 'They're just stories. Don't tell yourself the stories, stay with the feelings.'" Ultimately, both approaches may work to help alleviate feelings of depression. But you may want to know how your meditation teacher views depression and emerging trauma memories before you sign up for a long retreat with him or her.

Whether you meditate or not, going on retreat to a sacred place can have a healing effect on your emotional well-being. A recent study published in the *British Medical Journal* found that Indians with a variety of mental illnesses reduced their symptoms by 20 percent without any sort of treatment or required practice. They simply spent several weeks living at the Hindu temple of Muthuswamy in South India, which is thought to have restorative benefits for people suffering from mental conditions.[14]

Gratitude

According to Edward's teacher, Vipassana teacher and *Yoga Journal* columnist Phillip Moffitt, the cultivation of gratitude is a powerful form of mindfulness practice, "particularly for students who have depressive or self-defeating feelings and those with a reactive personality who habitually notice everything that's wrong with a situation."[15] Even in difficult situations, gratitude can be cultivated. Moffitt instructs his students to first acknowledge the difficulty, then find the gift. An example would be "I am angry in this moment, and I am grateful I have a mind which knows this is so and can deal with it."[16]

Finding the gift in the moment of sadness may not eradicate the sadness, but it may bring your emotional body back into balance. Recently, during a period of mourning, there were times when the pain was so acute I had to get down on the floor and cry, sometimes curling into myself and rocking like a child, sometimes lying still. Even in these deep releases of my grief, I consciously acknowledged my gratitude for my big heart and my enormous capacity to feel. Soon after acknowledging my gratitude, my grief abated and I could resume whatever activity the outpouring of emotion had interrupted. I felt emptied out, still sad, but also refreshed and awake to the gift of each moment, each breath.

When the Container Leaks — Major Depression and PTSD

In the early stages of her meditation practice, Rachel sat through anxious feelings and mental distractions that for many of us would have been intolerable. It is sometimes difficult to focus the mind when you are feeling anxious or depressed. According to psychiatrist Roy King, who for eight years ran the Outpatient Partial Hospitalization Program at Stanford University Hospital and incorporated Yoga asanas and meditation into his treatment, major depression impairs our ability to focus. During a major depressive episode, it is unlikely that focusing on the breath or the changing thoughts in the mind will be effective. In fact, trying to follow the thoughts may make the depression worse. People suffering from depression are highly distractible, says King.

In working with depressed patients, King gives them a lot of encouragement so that they will not become frustrated and give up. People suffering from depression "have a tendency to go back to negative thoughts." King coaches his patients to "observe the negative thought when it comes in and then let it go." When a patient is unable to do this, King suggests an open-eyed form of concentration on an object. In his work with patients suffering from depression, he might use an orange—something specific and concrete. This form of focused attention on an object in the environment can create a sense of one-pointed awareness (*Dharana*), and may help center the mind when it is too busy or distracted to observe its own thoughts.

Sitting in meditation, paying attention to the thoughts and feelings that arise, may occasionally bring up memories, flashbacks to traumatic events, and the emotions that attend those events. "Spiritual work," says John Tarrant, "brings us down to the foundations of life before it lets us rise." Boston psychotherapist and trauma specialist Deirdre Fay, who incorporates meditation practices and Yoga philosophy in the workshops she teaches internationally, uses both mindfulness and concentration techniques with men and women who have histories of traumatizing abuse. Her goal, she says, is "to give people more skills to master their life, so that they can free themselves of their history rather than be propelled by their history."

Sometimes a concentration technique will initiate a blissful state that for someone who has suffered from traumatizing sexual abuse may feel overwhelming, perhaps triggering memories of the original abuse. If this happens, Deirdre might encourage her client to switch to a mindfulness technique, in order to more clearly observe the thoughts and feelings aroused by the experience. For some severely traumatized individuals, whose boundaries are not clear, who lack a clear sense of self, "if they drop into regressive material, they can get lost there for days." Switching to a mindfulness technique can ground them again, and "keep them in their adult self, the part of them that has the resources and capacity to have a functioning life." Deirdre believes that even victims of trauma can be served by a technique that "builds the observing self and decreases identification with what's happening." In small, regulated doses—she recommends limiting mindfulness practice to three minutes to start—she says that her clients who practice mindfulness meditation can "learn to name and observe previous untamable thoughts and feelings and begin to feel more relaxed."

It is important to keep in mind that Deirdre's traumatized clients have her direct observation and support as they begin a meditation practice. I would not recommend even mindfulness meditation practice for someone who has been severely traumatized, unless you are practicing with the guidance of a psychotherapist trained to teach meditation. Even with support, there may be circumstances when the trauma is too stark, the pain too profound, the rage too pronounced, and the container still too weak to simply sit and observe the thoughts. In cases of severe trauma or major depression, it may be better not to sit in meditation, but to focus on strengthening the container by doing something physical, like Yoga asanas or some other form of physical exercise. "Meditation produces an inward-looking dynamic," says Janis Carter, the psychiatrist in Brisbane, Australia, who uses Yoga in her treatment of Vietnam veterans suffering from post-traumatic stress syndrome. "In depression, this dynamic is overdeveloped, and has become quite narcissistic. In my clinical experience, I have found meditation to be potentially quite dangerous with this population. With the asanas, practitioners move spontaneously into the meditative state, and that, in my opinion, is sufficient."

Active Meditation Techniques

There are other, more active meditation practices that engage the brain in ways that may be easier to practice for those who are recovering from trauma and major depression. For some, a long-term practice of observing the changing mind states may eventually create a compassionate container, enabling the meditator to witness his passing thoughts and feelings and not be retraumatized by old memories. But for others, particularly those suffering from major depression or PTSD, a practice that engages the mind fully with mantra, light, mudra, and/or breath may be a better way to begin. "If you ask someone who is suffering from major depression to sit down, be quiet, and watch the breath, they may go deeper into the depression," says senior Viniyoga teacher and author Gary Kraftsow.

He is not alone in recommending a more active meditation practice for people suffering from major depression. In fact, there is scientific

evidence suggesting that practices that use visualization actually activate a different part of the brain. According to Roy King and his colleague Ann Brownstone, research has shown that the sitting techniques
that use mantra or breath, what they call "aniconic" techniques, differ
from imagery-based meditations in terms of regional brain activity.[17] In
the first set of practices, brain scans have shown a reduction in the
occipital and parietal areas of the cortex, while more active practices
like the body scanning and relaxation exercises often done in Corpse
Pose (Shavasana) at the end of Yoga class and pleasing visualizations are
shown to activate the occipital cortex. The occipital cortex is the main
processing center for visual information, both what we actually see and
what we imagine. It is responsible for hypnogogic imagery, those drifting pictures we sometimes receive when we are about to fall asleep. Roy
King believes that meditation practices that involve focused imagery
activate these pleasant visualization processes while deactivating the
prefrontal cortex, thereby muting cognitions, anxious thoughts, and
obsessions.

Meditation techniques that take a person out of his self-fixation and
connect him with the energy that nurtures him may initially be more
beneficial than techniques that focus inward. If you suffer from major
depression or PTSD, rather than sitting, observing your mind states,
rather than inquiry into past trauma and causes, it may be more helpful
to use words and affirmations and images that take you beyond your sorrow into joy. Mantra chanting is one such technique that can put you in
contact with the potential for joy within you that may be masked by
your depression.

Mantra Chanting

Mantra chanting meditation helped Mary, a thirty-six-year-old elementary-school teacher in Boston who finally graduated from college when
she was thirty. Mary grew up in New York City, the only child of parents
who had little time for her childish needs. Her mother had been a
prima ballerina with a national company before Mary was born, and
when Mary was three, founded her own touring dance company. Her
father, a successful concert musician, was also often on the road, and
Mary was raised by a succession of nannies. Mary's parents paid little
attention to her minor accomplishments, and one or both of them were

usually away for the important events of her life. Though she had doting grandparents with whom she spent time, they couldn't fill the absence of her mother and father. When she was eleven, Mary got caught shoplifting a velvet clutch bag, high heels three sizes too big for her feet, and a bottle of expensive perfume from an exclusive department store. That caught her parents' attention and she was sent to boarding school. When Mary ran away for the second time, they allowed her to come home, began making strict rules about curfews, bedtimes, and homework, and occasionally stayed home to enforce them.

Mary matured early and received a lot of attention from boys. When she became pregnant at fifteen, her mother arranged the abortion. Soon after that, Mary ran away again, this time living on the streets for three weeks until one of her grandparents spotted her in the East Village and brought her home. When she returned, Mary escaped from the reality of her life at home through her abuse of drugs and alcohol. The psychiatrist she saw weekly thought she was depressed. But Mary didn't buy it. What she bought was transcendence—LSD, cocaine, and eventually heroin. Ironically, she began doing Yoga during this time in her life. "It was just part of the scene," she says. "It enhanced the effects of the cocaine."

For most of her life, Mary has yearned for connection, but the elders in her life were incapable of an intimate and loving connection with her. Her parents were too self-absorbed to show her the wonder of the universe. What they showed her was a wall of narcissism so thick that only "being bad" could penetrate it. The only time they interrupted their busy schedule was when she was in trouble. The only serious talks they had with her were when she was caught doing something wrong. To escape her suffering, she drank, smoked pot, and used cocaine. But she needed ever-increasing amounts to avoid her pain. Eventually, confined to a treatment center for five weeks when she was twenty-six, she learned a Kundalini chanting meditation technique that she says saved her life.

Mary found it difficult to sit on a meditation cushion for twenty minutes, observing her breath or paying attention to a mantra held in her mind, but she could chant mantras aloud for twenty minutes and she would feel better. The mantra-chanting meditation met her busy, unfocused mind with a plan. Her teacher offered her a practice that met her somersaulting thoughts with some Kundalini mental gymnastics—she was taught to focus on a series of mantras and hand movements while visualizing a sweep of white light through her mind.

You don't have to have suffered from the effects of drug and alcohol abuse to appreciate the natural high of Kundalini meditation practice. Alice, a massage therapist and Kundalini student whose mother died when she was eight, has had bouts of major depression for most of her life. Even now when she doesn't practice daily she is likely to feel depressed. "If I begin my day with a Kundalini meditation practice, I have more energy and usually feel pretty good no matter what problems arise."

There are a number of different Kundalini meditation techniques taught by Yogi Bhajan and the teachers he has trained. Many of them use breath, mudra, mantra, and visualization, techniques that keep the mind focused and engaged. The effect, however, is a vacation from the way we normally think, a respite from obsessive or negative thoughts. One feels refreshed and relaxed and yet energized after a Kundalini meditation practice. Most often, Kundalini meditation techniques are used in the context of a larger practice that includes physical exercises, breathing exercises, and chanting. It is important to learn Kundalini yoga from a qualified Kundalini teacher. Energy-based meditation techniques like Kundalini and those taught in the Tantric tradition can be too energizing for certain systems, particularly for someone who is bipolar or suffers from other psychiatric disorders, like schizophrenia. But for most people suffering from depression, if you learn and practice them with an experienced teacher, you will benefit from these energizing techniques.

Sanskrit scholar and Ayurvedic doctor Swami Sivananda Sarasvati teaches Yoga in Rhode Island. Another practitioner referred a young man named Jim, who suffered from intense anxiety and major depression, to Swami Sivananda, because Jim did not want to take medication. He hated his job in a military-related industry and obsessed about it constantly. Swami Sivananda recognized that Jim was too agitated to sit with his eyes closed in meditation, so he invited Jim, who was very conservative, to attend the fire ceremony he conducts at 6:00 every morning. The ceremony, which lasts about forty-five minutes, includes chanting and a twenty-minute active meditation. Jim loved the chanting, which helped calm and focus his mind. Midway through the ceremony, there is a *tratak* meditation in which the participants gaze at the fire. This active form of concentrated meditation worked well for Jim. According to Swami, in six months he was happy. He quit his loathsome job, found another more to his liking, and for the first time in years he has a girlfriend.

Guided Visualizations

Guided visualizations are a kind of meditation practice that can help with clinging thoughts, particularly for those experiencing the recurring flashbacks from a traumatic episode. Psychotherapist Kirsten Trabbic Michels, a Yoga teacher and Phoenix Rising Yoga Therapist, used guided visualizations in her work with Vietnam vets in a VA hospital in Maryland. She says that some combat veterans felt so unsafe in the world that trying to imagine a safe place during a guided visualization, while practicing in a group, would increase their anxiety level. "Relaxing for some vets," she says, "could actually allow the anxiety that had been contained, by whatever defense mechanism they were using, to rise to the surface. Their eyes would pop open, they would start moving around, and sometimes people would just sit up." On the other hand, when she worked with a vet individually and they talked first with eyes open about an image of safety, she was then able to guide him into a meditation with eyes closed, after which his anxiety lessened. For some vets, says Kirsten, "the safest imaginable place might be a cave in the middle of nowhere, hiding with his gun."

There are numerous New Age guided visualizations available on audiotape and CD, some of which are based on Yoga, that can quiet the negative self-talk and lift the spirits. At the end of Yoga class, I often lead a self-healing guided visualization. Based on the principles of Yoga philosophy, the visualization invites students to use the innate healing energy that they have uncovered with their practice to heal areas in their lives that may be out of balance. After class, students often tell me that not only do they feel both relaxed and refreshed, but they also feel empowered to heal themselves.

Spirit Dancing

If we stretch the definition of meditation to include spiritual practices that create a heightened state of awareness, then certainly dance must be included. For thousands of years, until they were banned in 1947, the *devadasi,* the temple dancers in India, honored the deities in their deeply meditative dancing that we in the West have come to know as Classical Indian dance. The Sufis understood the power of movement and dance, as did many indigenous cultures around the world. Lately, Yoga Dance and Trance Dance have become popular forms that combine spiritual intention with dance. Though there's been little research to document the effect of this kind of dance, practitioners tell stories about their recovery from depression through this form of mindful movement.

Peggy Schjeldahl has led Kripalu DansKinetics for eleven years. Unlike most other forms of dance, it's not step-oriented, but rather it's led as a spiritual practice with the intention of full self-expression through creative movement. Peggy's own recovery from depression has been facilitated by her practice of DansKinetics. A Kripalu DansKinetics class begins and ends with meditation. It incorporates Yoga stretches and aerobic movement. When practiced with intention and awareness, the fast-motion aerobic dancing has the capacity to lift you out of negative self-talk and into an elevated state of awareness. It's in the free-dance portions of the class where, says Peggy, "your spirit emerges. It brings an immediate feeling of joy, especially when practiced in the company of others."

Some people have found a heightened state of awareness and greater happiness from other forms of physical exercise, like running, biking, and weight training, when practiced with awareness and intention. When you practice Yoga with compassion, developing the habit of listening to your body and staying present to your experience in the moment, then you can take that awareness into any activity you enjoy—throwing pots on a wheel, playing the piano, writing poetry, gardening, long-distance running, swimming. Anything you love to do can become your practice as long as you bring the principles of self-acceptance and Witness Consciousness to your actions. When practiced consciously and with intention, you will gain a whole new level of satisfaction from your favorite activities.

Whatever the source of your depression and whatever its nature, there is a meditation technique that benefits you and allows you to step away from your depressive symptoms. At first, your respite may be only for the length of your practice, but with time you will find the feeling of serenity moving with you off your cushion and into your daily life.

yoga experience

To learn any of the meditation techniques discussed in this chapter, it is important to find a qualified teacher. Sometimes as you sit using any of the contemplative techniques, troubling thoughts may come or difficult emotions may arise. A teacher can answer your questions and ground you in your practice so that you can sit gently with the unexpected.

This meditation experience is called *karuna,* which in both Sanskrit and Pali means compassion. It is a wonderful technique, no matter your state of mind. How, even in our deepest depression or in the midst of a panic attack, can we find compassion for ourselves? The traditional Buddhist texts suggest two simple phrases to cultivate the state of compassion—*May I be free from suffering. May I find peace.* At first, as you repeat these phrases, they may feel hollow, especially if you are suffering right now from depression. Vipassana teacher and author Sharon Salzberg suggests that you modify the phrases so that they have meaning for you. "Sometimes," she says, "people feel more comfortable using a phrase that asks for a more loving acceptance of pain, rather than freedom from pain."[18] Find a phrase you can use with intention, and the effect will be cumulative and profound. In this meditation, by changing the pronoun to the second person, you offer compassion to others as well as yourself. Sometimes, when we're feeling depressed, it is hard to come out of ourselves, hard to see that there are people around us who may be suffering, too. Practicing karuna meditation can help break the grip of our self-absorbed, obsessive thoughts so that we are awake to compassion for ourselves and others.

Sometimes the darkness may feel so overwhelming that we forget even the memory of light. But when we bring compassion into the dark, we realize that we are not alone there. All human beings suffer. It is part of the human condition. In fact, says author and theologian Mathew Fox, suffering is "the heartbeat of the universe." Our suffering is both intimate—ours alone—and communal, connecting us with others, enlarging our capacity to feel compassion. When we practice karuna we grow our compassion, even in the darkness. The heart softens and the mind is soothed.

It is wonderful to practice this technique at the end of seated meditation, or you can do it by itself, perhaps in bed, before you fall asleep or when you first awaken before you rise to begin your day.

Begin in either a comfortable seated position with the spine erect, or lying on your back. Allow your eyes to close. If you are practicing this technique by itself, you might wish to take ten long Ocean-Sounding Victory Breaths (Ujjayi), inhaling and exhaling slowly through the nostrils, slightly constricting the back of the throat so that you make the wavelike sound of the ocean.

Now bring into your mind someone still alive who has offered you unconditional regard, someone whose love you can feel. Perhaps this person is suffering now, perhaps not. As human beings, we all face great physical pain or mental suffering in our lives. If your loved one isn't suffering now, he will be at some time in the future. See his or her face shining in your imagination. Continuing to breathe slowly and deeply, breathe in with the words *May you be free from suffering.* Breathe out with the words *May you find peace.* Feel that person's regard for you and send them compassion, repeating the phrases several times.

Now it is time to offer the same compassion to yourself. Repeat the phrases, using a long, slow inhalation and exhalation, changing the pronoun to "I." Acknowledge the suffering you have felt and the suffering you may have caused others as you continue to breathe and offer yourself compassion. Without any judgment, hold yourself as you would your beloved in your heart and offer yourself compassion and forgiveness. *May I be free from suffering. May I find peace.*

If you feel the compassion dissolving into fear or grief or some other disturbing mental state, do not judge yourself. Accept your humanness and acknowledge your heart—how you have the capacity to feel *all* your emotions. Come back to your breath, to Three-Part Yogic Breathing (*Dirga*), also adding the Ocean-Sounding Victory Breath if you wish. Fill yourself with the sound of your breath. Let the breath be like a soothing lullaby to yourself. Fill your lungs with breath until there is no more room, then exhale completely, so that you are completely empty and ready to receive. Do this several times. And if you feel calmer, resume your karuna practice.

Bring into your mind a person for whom your feelings are neutral. Imagine that person as you repeat the phrases again, returning to the use of "you." *May you be free from suffering. May you find peace.*

If at any time you find yourself despairing, accept where you are without judgment and drop the practice, returning to the pranayama breathing exercises as described earlier.

Now think about someone with whom you are having some difficulty. Do not begin with someone who has caused you deep distress in your life or someone you are not ready to forgive. Repeat the phrases silently, using the breath and imagining this person's face as you offer her or him compassion. *May you be free from suffering. May you find peace.*

Feel how spacious your mind is now. Feel how much more room there is in your heart. From this place of expanded consciousness, imagine you are looking down upon the town in which you live. Repeat the phrases silently, using deep inhalations and exhalations, several times, sending compassion to all who live in your town. *May you be free from suffering. May you find peace.*

Now feel how much bigger your heart has grown, and imagine you are looking down at the state in which you live. Repeat the phrases silently, sending compassion to all who live in your state. *May you be free from suffering. May you find peace.*

Continue to expand your view, imagining your country. Repeat the phrases silently, breathing consciously and sending compassion to all who live in your country. *May you be free from suffering. May you find peace.*

Bring into your mind an area of trouble on the planet. Feel your compassion extending to those in conflict. Repeat the phrases silently, sending compassion to all who live in this troubled area of the world. *May you be free from suffering. May you find peace.*

Now imagine the earth spinning on its axis. Repeat the phrases silently, sending compassion to all beings on the planet, to all beings in the universe, to those in their bodies and those who have left their bodies and those who have yet to come. *May all beings be free from suffering. May all beings find peace.*

When you have sent compassion to all, take several moments to breathe deeply, feeling your inner connection to all beings. Then offer compassion once again to yourself. *May I be free from suffering. May I find peace.* Slowly, when you are ready, you may open your eyes, or if it's bedtime, have a good night's sleep. You can do this meditation completely or in parts—for example, offering compassion to yourself and to just one other. You can also use the phrases throughout the day to counteract negative self-talk or obsessive thoughts. Whether you are practicing on your meditation cushion or while standing in line at the grocery store, the effect of offering compassion to yourself and others will create more space in your mind and heart. As you continue to practice, you will feel lighter, less constricted, and the light of compassion will shine through the darkness.[19]

grief in the tissues— releasing trauma

Go in and in.
        Be the space
between two cells,
        the vast, resounding
silence in which
        spirit dwells . . .
Go in and in
        and turn away from
nothing that you find.

—DANNA FAULDS, from "Go In and In," *Go In and In*[1]

Many Yoga masters, Yoga therapists, and somatic psychologists believe that everything we've ever experienced is stored in the body.[2] Even when traumatic memory is repressed, the body remembers. International Yoga teacher and clinical psychologist Richard Miller sees depression as a somatic-based problem that has settled into the tissues. He says depressed people need bodywork. "Yoga is an exquisite form of body work that eliminates the residue that has become lodged in the tissue."[3] Lama Palden Drolma, a psychotherapist and founding teacher of the Sukhasiddhi Foundation, agrees. "Yogic practices," she says, "bring us to a state of ripeness. They purify the energy channels for the free flow of *prana* [life force, energy]. In the process, the sludge is brought to the surface. It's like cleaning the sewers. The psychological and emotional obstacles get flushed to the surface." When you practice every day, the ordinary losses you have faced in your life, losses that have become "lodged in the tissue," begin to dissolve. Eventually, even the most traumatic of experiences may be released.

When a Yoga class moves slowly and students are guided to stay focused on the breath and the sensations in their bodies while they hold a pose, perhaps longer than their self-limiting fears might otherwise allow, long-buried memory can sometimes become conscious, and feelings that have been repressed can surface. This deep psychological work comes slowly. Unless specifically guided, the deepest cleansing rarely occurs spontaneously in the first stages of Yoga practice, but rather when the student is more experienced and comfortable with longer holdings of a posture. Deep releases, be they physical, energetic, or emotional, come "when the student is ready," says Richard Miller.

The Holding Environment

However, it's always possible that the *teacher* leading the class may not be ready. A possible problem arises when the Yoga instructor, out of fear or inexperience, or even a misguided caring for the student, seeks to limit the student's experience. In so doing, the situation may duplicate the original traumatic experience in which the student may have felt unheard or even shamed. Although this duplication, within the context of a Yoga class where the teacher is well-intentioned and caring, may have within it the seeds for healing from the original wound, it can be retraumatizing. Therefore, it's important that you find a teacher you trust and a class where you feel safe. Psychologists call this a "holding environment." It's the place we feel safe enough to do emotional work. In the context of a Yoga class, you want to be free to experience what is most authentic about yourself, without the risk of feeling judged.

Here we are talking about the more ordinary losses we've faced in the course of our lives, losses that may not have been processed and released from the body. However, if you suffer from post-traumatic stress syndrome resulting from violence or torture, you need to exercise caution. For you, safety and trust are essential, and you may want to work individually with a qualified Yoga therapist and mental health practitioner. Maryanna Eckberg, Ph.D., a somatic psychotherapist who specializes in working with survivors of political torture, says that when an individual has suffered severe and violent abuse, "approaches that subscribe to cathartic release risk retraumatizing the patient."[4]

A "holding environment" can take the form of a relationship with a therapist, a Yoga class, or even a community of loving friends. "No one will go to the depths of terror alone," says Lama Palden Drolma. "The experience of not trusting the universe arises in our families so that by having a loving presence in our *sangha* [community] or therapy, someone to hold the space while we're in turmoil, we begin again to trust the world." How do we learn to trust when the neural patterns that establish the template for our relationships throughout our lives were formed in the limbic (feeling) brain based on the kind of care we received early in life? "When a limbic connection [important relationship] has established a neural pattern," say the authors of *A General Theory of Love*, "it takes a limbic connection to revise it."[5] Reading self-help books does not alter neural pathways. We must experience the change in our bodies and in the limbic soup where our attachments were first formed.

Later in this chapter, we'll talk about Yoga therapies that can safely, in a guided setting, facilitate the release of repressed emotion for most people. Though these therapies are not recommended for survivors of violent sexual abuse or torture unless accompanied by psychotherapy, most of us can feel tremendous relief when we involve the body in the release of emotion through Hatha Yoga. Occasionally, when the student is ready, these releases happen spontaneously, as was the case with Wendy, who had been practicing Yoga daily for two years when she experienced a major transformation through her practice.

Wendy

Wendy, at forty-five, looks as though she's in her mid-thirties. She's a small, attractive woman with dark brown hair stylishly framing a heart-shaped face and soft brown eyes that aren't afraid to meet yours when you speak with her, and many people do. Wendy is a clinical social worker who currently works for an agency specializing in addictions and maintains a small private practice in Tucson. Though she had experienced several rounds of psychotherapy over the years and was medicated for depression when I met her, there were more good days than bad. Still, every so often the blanket of dysthymia enshrouded her despite the antidepressant. Mostly she blamed her depressed mood on her inability to sustain a loving, intimate relationship. She couldn't understand why, when she so yearned for love in her life, her relationships didn't last. She believed that the problem might be related to her unwillingness to accept and express anger directly. Despite a few months in a Gestalt therapy group, in situations where most people would get angry, Wendy felt sad.

In psychological terms, depression is often conceptualized as anger toward the self. Since in Wendy's family it was not okay for her to express the normal frustrations and angry feelings a child has toward her parents, her anger turned inward. When someone close to Wendy expressed anger toward her, a kind of fog would settle around her, and she felt herself "numbing out." The next thing she knew, that numbness seemed to spread into all areas of her life. This happened when she was married to another therapist and living in Cincinnati. Her husband, whom in retrospect she would see as possessive and controlling, would sometimes rage at her, often because he felt her attention was elsewhere. When this occurred, Wendy withdrew even further, berating herself for her lack of feeling.

Wendy felt that it was her inability to deal with her negative feelings toward her husband, in the face of his rage, that led to her first major depression. The activities she enjoyed no longer interested her. She lost her motivation to exercise at the gym or ride her bike and often overate, bingeing on carbohydrates. As a result, she gained weight, which made her feel even worse about herself. She saw herself as undesirable and lost interest in sex. At work, she was less attentive in her sessions. "I was totally self-absorbed," she told me. "I forgot staff meetings, screwed up insurance forms, double-scheduled. When I missed an appointment two weeks in a row, I put in my resignation before they fired me." It took her two more years to end her marriage.

When the divorce was final, she became even more depressed and entered a series of sexual relationships that quickly dissolved. At the beginning of each relationship, she felt happy and reengaged enthusiastically with life. But no matter how good her partner looked on paper, or how well he pleased her in bed, her heart did not sustain the engagement. Often she felt the nicer someone was to her, the more appropriate the match, the harder it was to love him. She was most attracted to bullies who pushed past her boundaries because they "loved me so much."

Several years ago, Wendy moved to Arizona in the hope that she would feel better in a city where the chamber of commerce claims 362 days of sunshine a year. And she did for a while. But then the pattern of withdrawal began to repeat itself in a series of short-term relationships from which she was always the one to leave. When I met her, she was functioning well as a therapist, but there were sunny mornings when she woke up under a blanket of depression that dulled her senses. And she wanted the intimacy of a loving relationship with someone who didn't bully her. "Trouble is," she told me, "I'm never attracted to the 'nice guys.'"

Most of the time, her social mask was that of a well-put-together, organized, compassionate woman, and it fit her so well that, when she was at work, or swimming laps, or taking salsa lessons, she thought the depression was gone. But alone at night, she often drank several glasses of wine and microwaved a bag or two of popcorn. Then she would pass out in her chair and stumble into bed at 3:00 A.M., the day's makeup smearing her face, popcorn stuck in her teeth.

One day, while sitting in her dentist's waiting room, Wendy read an article I'd written for *Psychology Today* about Yoga's potential to alleviate depression. She remembered that she'd seen my name on a flyer at the Tucson Racquet and Fitness Club, where I teach early-morning Yoga classes and where she swims. Seven in the morning was early for Wendy to be out of bed in the company of others, and she brought a thermal mug of coffee to her first Yoga class. We joked about that. I suggested that she might not want to drink a stimulant while trying to relax and that the Yoga itself would energize her for the day.

I remember that first class, because Wendy couldn't seem to sit still during the centering meditation. She fidgeted with her Velcro wristbands and kept opening her eyes to see what everyone else was doing. Because I allow the class to be in their bodies in a way that feels comfortable, I let Wendy find her way through her first Yoga experience, with only gentle reminders to the whole class to breathe long, deep breaths through the nostrils and to practice, when comfortable, with the eyes closed. During the relaxation Wendy stared at the ceiling tiles, but her breath was even and slow, much calmer than when she'd begun the class.

After the class, I asked her how she felt. Based on her developed biceps and small, fit body, I imagined she was an athlete, accustomed to more aerobic activity, and that she might have been bored. "I loved it," she said, her eyes bright. She thanked me for the class and told me that she was a therapist suffering from depression, and asked if we might have coffee to talk a little more about Yoga.

"Coffee?"

"Okay, tea. *Black* tea."

Mostly what we talked about that day was Wendy—her failed relationships, her feeling that, as a therapist, she was a fraud because she felt lousy so much of the time, her hope that Yoga would help. I pointed to her untouched coffee mug, which sat beside her cup of tea. "Maybe it already has."

After that first day, Wendy stopped fidgeting and attended Yoga class regularly without her mug of coffee. Sometimes when I entered the room, Wendy was already there, down on her knees in Child Pose. I would see her bent head and wonder if she was suffering. Months later, she told me that in the beginning, when she went into Child Pose (*garbasana*) resting with her hips on her heels and her forehead on the mat, she would occasionally find herself crying "for no good reason." The Yogic understanding of Wendy's experience might be described in terms of the sheaths (*koshas*).

The Postclassical Yoga texts describe five *koshas,* or sheaths, each one enveloping the other. In simplest and inapproximate terms, the five sheaths equate to the physical body, the prana or energy body, the mind body, the understanding body, and the bliss body, where the small self comes in union with the Absolute. From our life experiences, we accumulate stored impressions (*samskaras*) in the sheaths, which can prevent us from experiencing life without preconceived limits. Through Yogic practices we have the opportunity to release these stored impressions, purifying the sheaths. These releases may not necessarily have thoughts and words attached to them, especially if the impressions, or samskaras, are formed through patterns of relationships with significant others, usually parents, before the acquisition of language.

So perhaps Wendy was simply releasing from the physical body or the energy body when she went into Child Pose, peeling another layer of the onion, purifying, in the process of "ripening," so that deeper releases would soon be possible. When Wendy's tears came, she said that afterward she mostly felt comforted, as though she were nurturing herself.

Sometimes, as a result of our practice, layers of armoring are slowly stripped away and, in Yogic terms, the five sheaths (koshas) are gradually purified. The process is so slow that we're not usually aware of this new ability to face our feelings until we are in a disturbing situation and find ourselves responding differently. Often the first indication may be that we feel genuine feelings of warmth toward our fellow practitioners and our Yoga teacher at the end of class. This may extend into our ordinary routine and into our interactions with others off the mat.

Though I often guide my students to respond with equanimity and awareness to the sensations in their bodies, to cultivate a state of mind that allows them to witness the sensations that arise in their physical and emotional bodies without judgment, this doesn't mean that I am suggesting that they feel less. In fact, it has been my experience that after Yoga practice, I can truly feel more. A Scandinavian study conducted several years ago explains why this might be true. Brain waves were measured before and after a two-hour Yoga class. Not only was there a 40 percent increase in alpha waves, which indicates that the mind is more deeply relaxed, but theta waves increased by 40 percent as well, indicating better access to emotion, memory, and the unconscious.[6]

Phoenix Rising Yoga Therapy founder Michael Lee noted this same effect in his work with troubled adolescents at a residential school for teenagers with emotionally based behavior problems. "Several of the therapists working with the students commented favorably on the work I was doing with them. After receiving a session or a class, students often opened up and were more inclined to share their whole story rather than just the chosen bits and pieces."[7] I've observed a similar phenomenon at the juvenile detention center in Tucson, where I volunteer. When I ask them how they're feeling in their physical bodies before the class begins, I often get a one-word answer, like "fine," sometimes in a belligerent tone of voice. By the end of the class, they are much more responsive and willing to share their feelings.

Over the fifteen years that I've been practicing Yoga daily, my own numbness has dissolved so that I feel more grief, not less. But also more joy. The difference is that I am secure in the knowledge that everything changes. I know that to cling and hold on to that which brings me joy (*raga*), or to try to avoid that which I find distasteful (*dvesha*), only restricts my ability to stay open to receive what life brings. What we are cultivating in our steady practice of Yoga is what the ancient scriptures refer to as detachment. This doesn't mean we stop feeling. What it means is that we no longer identify with our thoughts and our feelings, just as we don't identify with our house or our car or the way we earn our living. It means a consistent recognition that "I am not my house, my car, my job, my sadness, my anger, my annoyance," but rather, "I am conscious of all of these things."

Two years passed with Wendy practicing daily, sometimes using a videotape to guide her home session between scheduled classes, sometimes practicing on her own. She frequently expressed her gratitude for the ways in which Yoga was changing her life. "I can't remember the last time I felt the fog settling in," she told me. She was free of medication and was feeling positive about her community of friends and her work. She still longed for an intimate relationship, but despite the lack of one, she was happy with her life.

Then one day after class, Wendy told me that she wanted to discuss something that had come up for her during her home practice. In her therapy, she had recently begun looking at the "trauma bond" that had developed as a result of "my mother's colonization of my body." Jan Hindman was the first to use the term "trauma bond" to refer to the confusing bond that develops between the adult perpetrator of sexual abuse and the child victim, a bond that often affects the victim's intimate relationships throughout her life.[8] According to psychologist George Goldman, formerly Clinical Director of the Southern Arizona Center Against Sexual Assault (SACASA), "The trauma bond describes a process in which a young victim, who is already attached to the perpetrator, who already feels an instinctive dependence on the perpetrator, now has to integrate an assault into the fabric of the relationship. The significant and traumatic consequences are imprinted and may well remain throughout the victim's life, manifesting in various ways, which have to do with dependency, trust, and sexual response."

Current developments in neuroscience support trauma bond theory. Research shows that our earliest attachments establish neural pathways through our limbic brains that determine our adult attractions and attachments. For example, a woman with an alcoholic parent may not understand why, despite her attempts to date nonalcoholic men, she is continually drawn to the drunk at the bar. Psychiatrist Thomas Lewis, M.D., coauthor of the book *The General Theory of Love*, calls these patterns of attraction "faulty limbic attractors."[9] These limbic sparks determine why we light up when the wrong kind of partner approaches us, why we don't even notice the more suitable partner next door.

According to Wendy, her trauma bond was not the result of conscious sexual abuse on her mother's part, but rather her mother's panicked response to Wendy's failure to move her bowels in infancy. Wendy was the firstborn, and as such, her twenty-year-old mother wanted her to be the perfect reflection of her ability to mother. To her, perfection meant daily bowel movements and an extremely early toilet training. It also meant that expressions of anger weren't tolerated in Wendy's house. From infancy until a younger sibling was born when Wendy was nine, her mother, often with her father's assistance, helped Wendy's body to function properly, through a combination of daily doses of laxatives and regular enemas, administered with expressions of love and concern. The effect of her mother's control of her bodily functions and the repeated invasion of the enema, combined with her parents' insistence that she not display her anger, was a setup for a passive response to external force. Wendy learned to internalize her anger rather than express it.

It was also a setup for the trauma bond. For the enema, much as she despised it, was the way in which Wendy felt loved by her normally undemonstrative mother. According to psychologist and attachment theorist Patricia Critterden, when a mother is abusive or coercive with a loving expression, "the child then learns to associate a positive expression of feeling with a negative experience. When he later meets a peer or a potential lover, he will misinterpret positive expressions of feeling. He will assume that people who appear to be nice are being coercive."[10] This might be one of the reasons Wendy was having a difficult time sustaining a committed, long-term relationship.

Another reason for Wendy's difficulties could be how young she was when she separated from her mother. "There is a point in life," says

Richard Miller, "when the child is forced to choose separation over annihilation." Wendy was an infant when she withdrew from an over-controlling mother. How then, as an adult, could she possibly trust the universe enough to merge with another when her earliest experience of merging with her mother annihilated her physical boundaries? For satis-factory intimacy to occur, there must be, according to Buddhist theorist and psychoanalyst Mark Epstein, a temporary "surrender of ego bound-aries" and a "merging of the kind that characterizes all forms of love."[11] Wendy became so protective of her boundaries, she was unable to achieve that essential dissolution of self so necessary in love.

But that didn't stop her from yearning for that merger, that dissolu-tion of self. And she sometimes achieved it with one of her lovers, bul-lies attracted to the challenge of her boundaries who, time after time, pushed through them. For Wendy, it was the only way she could feel. Not surprising since survivors of abusive childhoods, according to George Goldman, often duplicate the power disparity they had with the abusing parent in their adult intimate relationships.

Wendy had spent five years in therapy in her twenties and had never talked about the abuse. Though she remembered the experiences of her later childhood years, between the ages of six and nine, the memories were filed away, without any feelings attached. When a child's physical bound-aries have not been respected, the child feels shame, anger, humiliation, and hopelessness, none of which Wendy was permitted to express. The feelings, along with the memories, were buried for many of her adult years.

It's easy to see how the trauma bond might contribute to Wendy's difficulty in establishing what she says she most wants in her life—inti-macy and love in a long-term monogamous relationship. Secure attach-ment in adults rests on a foundation set in childhood in which a child is allowed to feel he's okay even when he's expressing the normal aggres-sion that children feel toward their parents. This was something Wendy was never permitted to do. The good news is that recent findings in the field of neuroscience show that those "faulty limbic attractors" laid down in childhood can be adjusted and that the trauma bond can be bro-ken. "The emotional parts of the brain," says Thomas Lewis, "remain quite plastic and amenable to change."[12]

Wendy had gained so much in her ability to nurture herself in her Yoga practice. Could Yoga help Wendy break through her compliance

and passivity and begin to live from a place of authenticity and wholeness? In Yoga class, Wendy felt an unspoken permission to live from her
most authentic self. She was guided to accept the thoughts and feelings
that arose in her practice, to breathe fully into the sensations she experienced in each pose, to find her most authentic expression of each posture. The messages she received in class were of self-acceptance and
love, and little by little she gave herself permission to own her feelings,
to live from a true place. It's that permission, that atmosphere of acceptance that one can find in a Yoga class, the "holding environment" itself,
that may begin to undo the damage. Wendy was lucky. Her therapist
provided the container of safety and acceptance that enabled her to
examine her darker emotions without feeling judged. And she had a
Yoga class where the "sludge" could rise to the surface in an atmosphere
of self-acceptance.

There are wonderful Yoga masters in other Hatha Yoga traditions
who might have given Wendy a prescription of postures to perform and
another list of poses to avoid in order to improve her mood, or at the
least to distract her from the symptoms of depression. My approach,
as a Kripalu teacher, is to encourage students to accept what is true
in the emotional body as well as the physical body. I tell my students
what my teachers have said to me—that the first step toward transformation is to accept where you are now, without judgment. "In order to
reach your destination," I sometimes say in class, "you have to first
locate yourself on the map. Everything you need to reach that destination is already inside you." This kind of talk, which we might call the
language of self-acceptance, allows a student to begin practicing compassion toward himself, accepting even those things about himself he
most wishes to change. The words I speak in Yoga class have a direct
effect on my students' experience in a posture and my own fulfillment as
a teacher.

I believe that it was that growing acceptance that allowed Wendy
to tell me about an experience she had at home on her Yoga mat while
in Plough Pose (*Halasana*).[13] (Plough Pose is done from Shoulderstand
with the legs stretched out over and away from your head and your
feet touching the floor. I don't recommend that you try this without a
teacher, but I want you to have a picture in your mind of what Wendy
was doing on her mat.) She had begun to cry. "It was like a baby sobbing,"

she told me. At first, Wendy had been frightened that she was losing control. But after her tears subsided, she felt so good that she welcomed the experience when it occurred the next day. "I was crying, but also watching myself cry, wondering where all the tears were coming from."

In fact, Wendy knew she had permission to cry. Most of my students, including Wendy, have seen me teaching with tears rolling down my face. I have often explained to students that crying can happen and we needn't be afraid. Sometimes it's just a release, another layer of tension peeling away. And sometimes there are particular emotions associated with the tears. But the practice itself will bring the emotional body back into balance.

As we learn to witness the rise and fall of the emotions, particularly when we are holding postures for an extended period of time, we are developing a kind of desensitization, so that we can see the events in our lives without the original feelings of confusion and terror attached. In Yoga, we call this Witness Consciousness or the Seer. Freud alluded to this Witness Consciousness when he said that the patient "must find the courage to direct his attention to the phenomena of his illness."[14] He also talked about the importance of "reconciliation with the repressed symptoms" and a "certain tolerance for the state of being ill." Reconciliation, tolerance, acceptance—these concepts are fundamental to Eastern philosophy, and to the Kripalu Yoga approach of being with what is authentic, even when it's painful.

According to Buddhist psychoanalyst Mark Epstein, there are those in the psychoanalytic field "who see the possibility of transformation of the infantile drives through the process of giving them access to consciousness."[15] He says that the Buddha's vision is that suffering is transformed not by avoiding it but by "changing the way we relate to it." He goes on to say, "Liberation from the Wheel of Life (*Samsara*), the chain of birth, death and rebirth, does not mean escape," but rather "clear perception of oneself, of the entire range of human experience."[16] This is *svadhyaya* again, "self-study," or as Swami Kripalu said, "self-observation without judgment."

Wendy was courageous, willing to take Plough Pose day after day, to hold the posture, to explore the feelings that arose, without judgment. Soon she began to believe that she was releasing old trauma stored in her body. When we experience trauma or loss and it is not fully acknowledged or accepted at the time of the experience, energy can be trapped in the body. "Whatever is refused," says Richard Miller, "leaves behind a residue." Yoga can provide a safe way to release this trapped energy, stored as tension in the body. We may have a physical symptom like chronic neck pain or a constriction in the chest or abdomen, something that mirrors in the physical body what is blocked in the emotional body. Or we may be free of symptoms and find the block only in the long holding of a posture.

Michael Lee describes his own cathartic release while he was living at Kripalu Center in the mid-eighties:

> One of my friends was using a wall to support me in the triangle posture on my right side when my body began to quiver uncontrollably. I witnessed an intense red-blue, burning sensation in my right hip and believed I had pressed into the posture as deeply as I could, feeling pain that wasn't really pain. My mind was shouting, "Get out of here! Stop now! Get on with it!" I was definitely at an edge between the known and safe and the unknown, unsafe territories of bodily existence. The escalating sensations in my right hip were becoming almost unbearable when my attention shifted from what was happening in my body to what was taking place in my attitude. I was becoming more and more agitated and wanted to release out of the posture. Placing his hand gently against my chest, my friend embraced my growing resistance by encouraging me to stay in the pose a while longer. His affirming presence made me feel safe and I surrendered again and again into what was happening in the moment, deepening my breath and simply witnessing the strange noises emanating from my mouth and my throat. The hot, fire-red burning seemed to pour out of my hip like a volcanic eruption. My whole body vibrated and I felt warm tears streaming down my face without my knowing why. My body began to feel very small as I re-experienced myself as an eight-year-old boy on a school playground about to be beaten up by a group of older boys. The terror of that frightened child permeated every cell of my being as I continued to release emotionally, feeling out of control, yet totally safe in the memory my body was releasing into consciousness.[17]

Not all releases in Yoga poses are accompanied by memory and emotion. Sometimes we tell ourselves a story about the release. Other times, there is no story, at least not a remembered one. For Wendy, at first, the release was purely physical. There were no memories attached to her crying episodes in Plough Pose.

Holding and Letting Go

I have had my own share of such episodes. A posture I have been practicing for years will suddenly release a flood of tears. Sometimes there's a story that goes along with the release, and sometimes it's simply a deep and profound letting go without any sort of knowing why. Vipassana meditation teacher, psychotherapist, and author Sylvia Boortstein has had similar experiences that have made her question the need to always know the story behind the release. "I've had some tremendous energy releases in sitting meditation and also in my Yoga practice. How do I know that these things didn't release themselves quite apart from my ever knowing what they were? Maybe they don't always have to come through the cognitive processes. Maybe I don't have to know that there was a time that my mother did 'this' or my father did 'that.' Maybe we get healed in other ways. We get better from flu without knowing exactly why or how."

For me, such a release first occurred in a long holding of Bridge Pose (*Setu Bandhasana*) in a workshop in the Main Chapel at Kripalu Center. Complete instructions for this pose are in the Yoga Experience at the end of this chapter. Bridge Pose is done while lying on the back with the feet planted hip-width apart and close to the buttocks. The pelvis and chest are raised toward the ceiling, but the neck and head are kept on the floor. Usually the hands are interlaced beneath the back, which draws the shoulder blades toward each other. Because the pelvis and chest areas are lifted and unprotected, this pose can bring up repressed emotion—fear is not uncommon, particularly in someone who may have been sexually traumatized.

No specific thoughts or feelings connected to events in my life rose with the long holding of Bridge Pose. Still, though, strong emotion was released. My thighs were shaking and, as directed, I tried to focus my awareness on the sensations in my body. I was feeling some strain in my quadriceps, and a strong urge to release the pose, when I suddenly experienced tremendous heat in my thighs and groin area and began to cry. These were not tears of pain, nor were they triggered by conscious memory. My body was simply letting go of something it had held on to for far too long.

After holding Bridge Pose for about ten minutes, I released the posture in a flood of sensations and spontaneous movements that had only slight resemblance to formal postures, until my body moved on its own into Child Pose. Even before I felt the teacher's gentle hand on my back, I was feeling a profound sense of peace, as though I were hovering in a state of grace. When I finally rejoined the class in a seated position for the final "Om," I felt a sense of contentment with life just as it was. I remember having the thought that I occasionally have after meditating—that if that state is what death will be like, then there's really no reason to fear it. What I'd achieved with that cathartic release of a cellular block (*samskara*) was a time-out for the rational mind, a few moments of deep rest, a glimpse of *samadhi*. This temporary state was just a taste of what it's like to be awake. Because we live our lives separated from the knowledge of who we really are, in those moments when we have released enough tension in our bodies to connect with our deepest source, we feel as though we're in an altered state. But you don't have to have such a dramatic release in order to feel awake. Sometimes, simply practicing with the intention of staying open to the life force (prana) or to all of your emotions, or to the divine, will connect you to that sense of wholeness.

There's another way to think about these moments of bliss. What if the intelligent awareness of bliss, *sat chit ananda,* is not an altered state but your natural state? Your practices on the mat, contracting and releasing, holding and letting go, can help you release the grief that trauma and loss have stored in your tissues. Eventually, through practice, those moments of samadhi expand until they are firmly established in your mind and you are living with your eyes wide open in a state that is called *sahaj samadhi*. This is your birthright—the natural state of the awakened one, the *jivan mukti*. "When Yoga works," Richard Miller said when I described my experience to him, "it moves us into our natural state of being, not an altered state, but the state in which we live before we give ourselves away, before we separate from ourselves."

Michael Lee describes a similar experience after his release from triangle posture. "Incredulously, the sensations passed almost as easily as they had come and I came out of the posture feeling very different. I felt stiller, quieter, suspended in a state of timelessness. I was very *present*— to the moment and to myself."[18]

It turned out that Wendy, too, took Child Pose for a long time (she had no idea how long) after her tears subsided and that she also felt at peace. "When I finally stop crying, I go into a tranquil state," she said. "It's like floating in amniotic fluid. I feel absolutely safe and protected. This might sound absurd, but it feels as though I'm floating in my therapist's womb."

In his book *Thoughts Without a Thinker*, Mark Epstein quotes Freud's description of this state of grace in similar terms. "Freud described the 'oceanic feeling' as the prototypical mystical experience: a sense of limitless and unbounded oneness with the universe that seeks the 'restoration of limitless narcissism' and the 'resurrection of infantile helplessness.'"[19] Not all meditative experiences are a return to the womb, but they often feel like a coming home to the "natural state" that Richard Miller describes, in which old patterns get broken up and released. Given the trauma that Wendy faced in infancy, a dose of "unbounded oneness" may have been exactly the healing experience she needed.

Psychotherapeutic Use of the Holding

There are specific therapies listed in the Resources section at the end of the book that make good therapeutic use of holding a Yoga posture, past the client's initial resistance and urge to let go. Physical tension and unconscious emotional holding can begin to be released in the safe, guided experience of working one-on-one with a Yoga therapist. But Wendy's releases were happening on her own at home, without the guidance of a teacher or Yoga therapist. After several cathartic releases while holding Plough Pose, Wendy began to associate Plough Pose with the position in which she must have been as an infant on the diaper-changing table when the enemas began.

Since Wendy's experience in Plough Pose seemed to be related to specific events in her life, she decided to take her mat into her next therapy session in order to work with her psychotherapist from the position of Plough. She chose to use Yoga as a way to experientially relive her painful experience in the presence of a trusted therapist, who could help her to process the emotions that surfaced.

Wendy came to believe that Plough Pose was triggering experiences of spontaneous regression to the preverbal state, when her abuse began. She had these experiences, not as a beginner on the mat, but when she was ready to witness the feelings and sensations that arose as a result of her practice. She had also developed enough equanimity and awareness (or Witness Consciousness) so that insight into her past wouldn't frighten her. She had the safe container of good therapy and had established a daily Yoga practice.

So was Wendy's lifelong struggle with depression in part the result of the energy knots (samskaras) that accumulated and lodged in her sheaths (koshas) each time she was traumatized by her mother? Her therapy session shed some light on the question. First, she felt empowered by her therapist's willingness to go along with an experiential session. "I feel that I'm setting the course of the therapy," she told me, "which I think for someone like me, who felt so overly controlled as a child, is really important." During the session, her therapist sat, not in his usual chair, but a little farther away to give Wendy space. At first, when she assumed Plough Pose, she was a little self-conscious about it, even though, in the position, she couldn't even see her therapist. She did not immediately burst into tears as she did when she practiced at home. But at a certain point she felt herself relaxing. She made a decision to let herself fully experience the emotions that surfaced in Plough Pose, without excluding her therapist from the process.

First, she became aware of the pressure in her neck, shoulders, and upper back. Soon she felt the choking feeling as well as a constriction in her chest. Then she noticed a pressure on her ankles and calves, "as though my mother's hands were pinning me down." Through dialogue with her therapist, she began to access her rage at being restrained and invaded. Soon she was kicking at the restraints and demanding that her mother let her go. Through the course of the session, her therapist kept her focused on what she was feeling and toward whom. At times, he role-played her mother, talking sometimes with the baby Wendy and sometimes with the adult Wendy. By the end of the session, Wendy had released more grief and had finally touched the thing she most feared, her anger at what had been done to her. And it was okay. In the safety of her therapist's office, on her Yoga mat, it was all okay.

What amazed Wendy was that, by the end of the session, she was feeling almost happy. "I felt grateful and warmly protected by my therapist. I held on to the leg of his empty chair and felt enormously supported by that. 'This is your chair,' I said again and again, feeling a deep sense of well-being." Maryanna Eckberg, Ph.D., noted this phenomenon in her work with survivors of political torture. "Frequently, the client's own unconscious will find balance, weaving back and forth on its own between the horror of the trauma and the healing resources which the deep recesses of the unconscious mind provide."[20]

It has been a year since Wendy spent a month crying whenever she entered Plough Pose, and she feels her life has been changed by the experience. For one thing, it's easier to be with her parents than it used to be. After expressing her anger on her mat and in her therapy sessions, Wendy was also able to talk to her parents about her feelings. "When I held the emotion inside, not even recognizing it as anger, for all those years, I felt stiff around them, around my mother, particularly. I was always on guard with her. My body would tense up in her presence. But since last year, I've been able to feel much more relaxed around them."

Wendy's softening toward her parents may have been the reason she experienced the most incredible change of all. After all those tears in Plough Pose and the deep work she was able to do with her therapist, Wendy feels that something opened inside her so that she was able to love in a new, less wary way. Soon after, she met a man she was attracted to and found herself falling in love with him. The miracle for her is that she has not yet withdrawn from him, even in situations where he's expressed his anger toward her. And several times she's been able to express her anger toward him. This time, she says, she's chosen someone who doesn't storm her boundaries. He doesn't have to. "I'm so much more open and receptive. The loving is better in all ways. Sometimes I think that I love the most incredible man there is, a man who is willing to surrender to me, as I surrender to him. But my therapist reminds me that it's me who has changed. 'It's you, Wendy,' he says."

Yoga Therapy

There are several "Yoga therapies" designed to accomplish the kind of transformation Wendy experienced. These therapies work with clients on an individual basis, using poses to access repressed emotion, with the Yoga therapist acting, along with the client, as witness to the experience. One of the first techniques to be developed that combines Yoga postures with active listening between client and Yoga therapist is Phoenix Rising Yoga Therapy (PRYT). Founder Michael Lee, quoted above, had been a student of Yogi Amrit Desai, who, in the early days of Kripalu Yoga, often guided long holdings of postures to access and release repressed emotions. Lee developed PRYT as a form of therapy in the years following his breakthrough in Triangle Pose. "One of the primary ways of speeding up our evolution as human beings," says Lee, "is to increase awareness, to become the witness, to observe oneself without being caught up in what one observes. The practice of Phoenix Rising Yoga Therapy is in part designed to facilitate this process. It also goes a step further. Through a dialogue process it seeks to put words to the observations of self." According to Lee, "The loving and nonjudgmental presence of the practitioner creates the sanctuary for such observations."

Bob Martynski, a massage therapist and Yoga practitioner in Milwaukee, is studying to become a Phoenix Rising Yoga Therapy practitioner because of the emotional breakthrough he experienced while holding a Yoga pose on his own. For years, Bob struggled with a debilitating depression that began in a childhood marred by family alcoholism, violence, and physical abuse. "I came across a picture of me at five, sitting on a brick wall in my grandfather's garden. My arms are clutched tightly across my chest, and I'm slumped forward. I have a very sad expression on my face, like I might be grieving a great loss, and there are dark spots below my eyes." Bob's memories of childhood are of shutting down, "of retreating inward, hiding, disappearing." In adulthood, Bob suffered from an anxiety-based depression so severe that it disrupted his education, his relationships, and his work life. In 1975, he had his first experience with Yoga when he taught himself breathing techniques that he read about in a magazine article about a Hollywood celebrity who had discovered the joys of Yoga. He noticed an immediate calming effect from Yogic Three-Part Breath (Dirga) and an energizing effect from Breath of Fire. He found a teacher in 1976 and began to practice regularly. However, his practice evoked thoughts and feelings that he was not prepared to handle. At that time, he says, "there weren't any teachers around prepared to guide me through my feelings. I began nearly two decades of dancing toward and away from my practice."

Yoga kept Bob's head above the darkness, and he "limped along for years with a weak practice that was just enough to sustain my spirit." Then, in 1996, he came across a picture of someone in Upward-Facing Bow (*Urdva Danurasana*), known in some Yoga traditions as Wheel Pose. "I became absolutely obsessed with that image, and a voice somewhere deep inside of me said I must learn that asana." The Wheel is perhaps the most difficult of all backbends and is also one of the most exhilarating. This is not a pose recommended for beginners, so I will not explain how to do it. But so that you can visualize what Bob was attempting to do, imagine your body draped backward over a large beach ball, then imagine that the beach ball were removed. For Bob, who had been practicing for twenty years by the time he began to prepare his body for this pose, learning the Wheel was "an incredible and slightly amusing adventure. I couldn't lift my body off the ground to save my life." After months of practice, he was finally able to arch his body upward from the floor, but it made him feel dizzy. More months of practice and the use of a prop called the Body Bridge enabled him to overcome his dizziness and spatial disorientation. When he finally accomplished the pose, arching his body into the proper form, he experienced a rush of heat and energy through the front of his body. "I felt like I had been turned into liquid fire," he says. "I began to sweat, then shake, not from fatigue but streaming energy. The sense of opening was tremendous." This posture initiated some major life changes for Bob. "It seemed to give me access to some hidden source of inner power." As he continued to practice the pose, his physical strength and inner resources seemed to increase. "I was able to quit a job I absolutely hated but had endured for almost eighteen years." That's when, after experiencing for himself the deep release available in the long holding of Wheel Pose, he decided to train to become a Phoenix Rising Yoga Therapist.

Though not specifically a "Yoga therapy," the Kripalu Yoga approach to self-discovery uses methodology to develop an individual's own Witness Consciousness during long holdings of postures so that if repressed feelings and thoughts become conscious, they do so in a mind grown more equanimous and self-aware, a mind less attached to the feelings evoked by the original trauma. Psychologist Rasmani Deborah Orth, longtime Kripalu program director and dean of the Kripalu faculty, says that in Kripalu Center's Self-Discovery Programs, "We spend time creating the context so there is a way for the participant to understand her or his experience of holding a posture. We discuss how to practice being present, so that the participant doesn't become overwhelmed or frightened by the experience and is able to relax into whatever arises on a physical or emotional level." Rasmani and the other Kripalu program directors talk about the experience of "riding the wave," observing the thoughts, feelings, and sensations that arise during the experience. "There is often the urge to jump off the wave," she says, "but if we stay on, we reach a point, an emotional peak or a physical peak. It may even be an unexpected point of silence. Sometimes in this moment, we experience an 'ah-ha,' a kind of insight. We connect with an energy that can take us beyond our habitual minds." During the holding, the participant stays present and cultivates Witness Consciousness and presence when he is coached with the words "breathe, relax, feel, watch, allow." In riding the wave, Rasmani says, it's helpful to "describe the experience in all its details, without labeling or having to understand why. Sometimes we make connections with our psychological history in the process, and other times there may simply be a release."

Guests at Kripalu Center who are about to experience their first long holding are sometimes concerned with physical pain they imagine they may encounter. The long holding is not designed to induce pain but rather a feeling of strong sensation in the body, the kind that disappears when the posture is released. "People are often surprised by how much strength they actually have," says Rasmani. "They feel a new connection to their energy and their life force—sometimes that feels like transcendence." This experience, like Wendy's after holding Plough Pose and mine after holding Bridge Pose, is not an altered experience but our *natural* state. The more we release those emotional and energetic blocks through our practices, the more freedom we will have to live from that place of unobstructed space, what the Yogis call *sukha,* or happiness.

For Wendy, the road back to building sufficient trust in the universe in order to sustain a loving relationship was not only the release of anger but her recognition that as an infant, she chose to protect herself by withdrawing, by withholding, by separating. It was within the context of the "holding environment," created in her therapy, that she was able to use Plough Pose to release at the deepest level the grief in her tissues, clearing the way for her to choose love over separation. At the time Wendy brought her Yoga mat into her therapist's office and assumed Plough Pose, her therapist was her mirror, her witness, and as such, was helping her develop her own Witness Consciousness. Eventually, if all goes well in her therapy, Wendy will be able to "take back the mirror," as Richard Miller puts it, and become a "holding environment for herself."

yoga experience

This experience is recommended for experienced Yoga practitioners, or beginners with the support of a qualified Yoga teacher or Yoga therapist. Remember, whatever comes up in your physical body and your emotional body, feel it fully, but also witness it with equanimity and awareness. Your partner will help you do this. It is important to create this experience with someone you trust, who can offer you support and unconditional acceptance as you move into unfamiliar territory in your physical body and your emotional body. This might be a psychotherapist, a holistic healer, a beloved intimate, or fellow Yoga practitioner and friend. Establish your partner's role in the process. She will be coaching you with words of acceptance.

First, warm up the body with easy stretching, or perhaps you and your partner can do some warm-ups and postures together. Then choose a posture you can hold for a long time without doing any damage to your body. You may choose Mountain Pose (*Tadasana*), as described in the Yoga Experience in Chapter Four, Bridge Pose (*Setu Bandhasana*), or any other posture in which you can remain steady and comfortable as you hold for several minutes.

Bridge Pose (Setu Bandhasana)

If you have chosen to take Bridge Pose as your holding posture, begin by lying on your back with your arms at your sides, palms facing down. Draw your feet up close to your buttocks and plant them on the floor, hip-width apart, so your knees face the ceiling. Your knees and feet should be parallel, with your knees directly over your ankles. Warm the body into the pose by pressing down into your feet and slowly lifting your pelvis toward the ceiling on an inhalation, then slowly release back down on an exhalation, staying aware of each vertebra as it touches the floor. Do this several times. When you feel ready, press all the way up

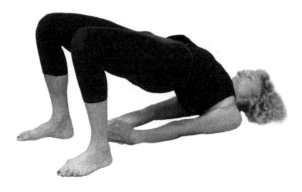

Bridge Pose (Setu Bandhasana)

and continue to breathe. Walk your shoulders toward each other beneath you, draw your arms away from your shoulders, and interlace your fingers with your little fingers touching your mat. Take long Ocean-Sounding Victory Breaths (ujjayi). Press into your big toes, and use isometric pressure between your knees. You can vary your arm position if you wish. You may use your palms to hold your hips up with your elbows resting on the mat. Or you may arch higher by reaching to hold your ankles with your hands.

Holding

Whichever posture you have chosen, move slowly and with awareness of all the sensations in your body into the holding of the pose. You may wish to hold it with some vigor at first, paying attention to the details of alignment. Then, as sensation begins to develop in your body, bring the breath to that place of strong sensation and your awareness will follow. Allow your mind to be totally absorbed in the physical sensations you are feeling. As thoughts rise to the surface of your mind, don't resist them. Watch what you are thinking, describe your thoughts to your partner, and then bring your attention back to the strongest sensation in your body. Likewise, as feelings come up, don't resist them. Describe them to your partner. Then return again to the physical sensations in your body.

In the beginning, your partner will use words that guide you to the physical sensations in your body—"Breathe, relax, feel, watch, allow"—saying them slowly, pausing between each word. These words can be repeated often, without variation, interspersed with words of encouragement like "You're doing great," "Beautiful holding," and so on. When you report your thoughts and feelings to your partner, she may repeat them back to you, as in, You: "I'm feeling a lot of heat in my shoulders." Partner: "You feel heat in your shoulders right now." Your partner will maintain this dialogue approach, repeating and affirming what you are describing in your physical body, your mind body, and your emotional body. She will resist the urge to interpret or analyze or judge. And she will repeatedly invite your awareness back to the sensations in your body.

As the physical sensations grow more intense, resist the first urge to release the posture, but tell your partner what you are feeling, how much you'd like to let go. She may repeat that desire back to you and encourage you to stay in the pose for a little while longer. Eventually you may find that you have gone beyond the physical discomfort in your body into sensations of pure light or heat in that area of your body. Or you may find that tears come, laughter comes, memory comes. Keep describing to your partner what you are feeling and thinking, without trying to label or analyze. Don't be afraid to make loud noises or to shout and say things you wouldn't want your mother to hear.

When you finally release the posture, do so slowly and move in *any* way your body tells you to move. Don't be afraid to listen to the wisdom of your body here, even if it takes you into movements you've never done before. Your body seeks homeostasis and will know what to do to bring you back into balance without your having to plan your movements in any way. Let your movements flow. It may look like Yoga or it may not. It may look like a dance or a crawl across the floor. The important thing is that you continue to take long, deep breaths through the nostrils and trust your body to guide you. When you feel complete, slowly come down to rest on your back in Corpse Pose or, if you prefer, in Child Pose. Take as long as you need, but at least five minutes. When you feel ready, come out of the resting pose and talk to your partner about what you're feeling. You may wish to take some time to write in your journal about your experience.[21]

Cautionary Note: This practice is not recommended for survivors of severe violence, torture, or sexual abuse without the support of a qualified psychotherapist trained in trauma intervention and somatic psychotherapy.

yoga on and off the mat

Here Amen
must be said
this crowning of words
which moves into hiding
and
peace
you great eyelid
closing on all unrest
your heavenly wreathe of lashes

You most gentle of all births.

—NELLY SACHS, "Someone"[1]

So here you are, having practiced and read and thought about the difference Yoga is beginning to make in your life. On the mat, it's easy. You hold a posture, breathing into the strong sensation, going deeper into an experience of being in your body in this moment, in Yoga, in union. When you release, you let go of what limits you, and you feel your expanded energy. You realize how little this energy pays attention to the boundaries of your physical body. In this moment you are aware of your wholeness. As your practice becomes steady and strong, you will have this awareness more and more in your daily life. But are there Yogic techniques you can practice off the mat that keep you from forgetting who you really are, that continue to clear the energy channels so that you are a vehicle for awakened prana? There are.

In the *Bhagavad Gita*, an ancient poem that is understood to be the philosophical foundation of Yoga, the charioteer Krishna, who later reveals himself to be God, counsels Arjuna (before a battle from which Arjuna shrinks) about the Yogic paths to enlightenment—Karma Yoga (the path of action without attachment), *Jnana* Yoga (the path of knowledge), and *Bhakti Yoga* (the path of love and devotion). By these different paths, the ancient Yogis acknowledged the differences in our constitutions.

The Jnana Path

> Wisdom springs from Yoga [practice]; Yoga derives from wisdom.
> For him who is dedicated to Yoga and wisdom, nothing is unattainable.
>
> —ANONYMOUS, "Song of the Divine," *Kurma-Purana*[2]

One way of remembering your wholeness is to approach Yoga through your intellect. Yoga need not be a mindless pursuit. While you may find that some individual practitioners have an anti-intellectual bias, Yoga truly honors the mind. Having come from a Yoga training in Gujarat, India, where I was steeped in practice, practice, practice, I remember the thrill I had upon first entering the Narayana Gurukula, a small ashram/school on a mountain in Ooty, the hill station town in the Indian state of Tamil Nadu. In the round, windowed reception room, the bookshelves were filled with literature from around the world. Not only were the great sages of Indian philosophy represented, but Western philosophers, poets, novelists, and scientists had their shelf space, too. Finally, I thought, I don't have to transcend the mind to find union in Yoga. In that reception room, while waiting to speak with Nitya Chaitanya Yati, the renowned Vedanta scholar with whom I'd come to study, I found total permission to use my mind as a vehicle for union with the divine.

The ancient Yogis acknowledged the differences in our constitutions. Some of us enjoy the pursuit of knowledge—we read, we discuss, we even debate, and we would not feel comfortable on a Yogic path if we believed we were supposed to abandon our critical-thinking mind in order to experience the union that is Yoga. If you love learning, perhaps the Jnana path is for you. You may be drawn to study more about Yoga philosophy or to learn Sanskrit. This is the path of the *Jnana* Yogi. In classical terms, the Jnana Yogi is one who finds liberation through the doorway of the intellect. Jnana Yoga is the Yoga of pure discrimination. It transcends the intellect through the intellect. If you find inspiration in literature, then you may find that your mood lifts simply from reading about the principles of Yoga.

Many students of Yoga finish their practice on the mat with a reading from an ancient text that inspires them, like the great sage Shankara's beautiful *Crest Jewel of Discrimination: Timeless Teachings on Nonduality,* or the *Bhagavad Gita,* or a book about practice like the *Yoga Sutras* or the *Hatha Yoga Pradipika.* Here's a passage I love from the *Crest Jewel of Discrimination.*

> The Atman is supreme, eternal, indivisible, pure consciousness, one without a second. It is the witness of the mind, intellect and other faculties. It is distinct from the gross and the subtle. It is the real I. It is the inner Being, the uttermost, everlasting joy . . .
>
> "You", "I", "this"—such ideas of separateness originate in the impurity of the mind. But when the vision of the Atman—the supreme, the absolute, the one without a second—shines forth in samadhi, then all sense of separateness vanishes, because the Reality has been firmly apprehended.[3]

Others may read from a contemporary book about Yoga philosophy and practice, like Stephen Cope's *Yoga and the Quest for the True Self* or Gary Kraftsow's *Yoga for Transformation.* Still others take inspiration from contemporary poetry by Mary Oliver or David Whyte or Jane Hirshfield. When I finish my own practice, I sometimes read from one of these poets or from the devotional poets like Rumi and Mirabai and Mechtild of Magdeburg, or from the wonderful translation by Anita Barrows and Joanna Macy of Rilke called *Rilke's Book of Hours: Love Poems to God.* Here's one of my favorite Rilke poems—it inspires a deeper opening and a sense of flow from my practice into my writing:

I Believe in All

I believe in all that has never yet been spoken.
I want to free what waits within me
so that what no one has dared wish for

may once again spring clear
without my contriving.

If this is arrogant, God, forgive me,
but this is what I need to say.
May what I do flow from me like a river,
no forcing and no holding back,
the way it is with children.

Then in these swelling and ebbing currents,
these deepening tides moving out, returning,
I will sing you as no one ever has,
streaming through widening channels
into the open sea.[4]

You may be drawn to read a portion from your own religious tradition—the weekly Torah or Bible portion or relevant passage from the Koran. Such reading brings you back from your practice into the world of the mind through the doorway of faith.

Faith

> Be ground. Be crumbled, so wildflowers will come up
> where you are. You've been
> stony for too many years. Try something different. Surrender.
>
> —RUMI, from "A Necessary Autumn Inside Each"[5]

In the early eighties, a blind study done in the San Francisco General Hospital's Coronary Care Unit involving 393 heart patients showed that patients who were prayed for had a better recovery rate from heart attack. Since then, there have been numerous studies documenting the importance of faith and prayer in recovery from illness and in maintaining optimal health and longevity. Dr. Harold Koenig, associate professor of medicine and psychiatry at Duke University, says many studies now show "intrinsic faith to be the most important factor in a patient's recovery from depression."[6] In fact, the U.S. government is currently funding a five-year study conducted by Dr. Koenig and his colleague, Dr. Diane Becker of Johns Hopkins University, in which women of color in the early stages of breast cancer are using prayer as part of their treatment. Studies have shown that people who maintain a strong religious faith experience less depression and anxiety and are less likely to commit suicide.

Does this mean that to be healthy you should go to church or temple every week? Not necessarily, though one study did show that regular church attendance increased longevity by 25 percent in men and 35 percent in women. What it means is that attending to your spiritual life, having a belief that sustains you, and expressing it in the company of others is good for your health. If you find sustenance in your faith, you may be a Bhakti Yogi.

The Bhakti Path

In

my soul

there is a temple, a shrine, a mosque, a church

where I kneel.

Prayer should bring us to an altar where no walls or names exist.

Is there not a region of love where the sovereignty is

illumined nothing,

where ecstasy gets poured into itself

and becomes

lost?

Where the wing is fully alive

but has no mind or

body?

In

my soul

there is a temple, a shrine, a mosque,

a church

that dissolve, that

dissolve in

God.

—RABIA, "In My Soul"[7]

Devotion (*bhakti*) is a path toward healing the heart. It is the union of loving devotion with faith. According to Yogic tradition, the *Bhakti* Yogi dedicates herself to the divine. "It is the only kind of attachment that does not reinforce the egoic personality and its destiny," says Yoga scholar and author Georg Feuerstein.[8] In the *Bhagavad Gita*, when Krishna counsels Arjuna about the three paths to enlightenment—Karma Yoga, Jnana Yoga, and Bhakti Yoga—he says that all three are legitimate routes to the ultimate goal of union, but that bhakti is the straightest, surest route for the ordinary person:

> All those who trust and love me,
> even the lowest of the low—
> prostitutes, beggars, slaves—
> will attain the ultimate goal.
>
> How much easier then for ordinary
> people, or for those with pure hearts.
> In this sad, vanishing world
> turn to me and find freedom.
>
> Concentrate your mind on me,
> fill your heart with my presence,
> love me, serve me, worship me,
> and you will attain me at last.[9]

Devotion is often expressed through chanting the names of God, which can have a harmonizing effect on the central nervous system. The subjective experience of even a few minutes of mantra chanting has always, for me, been both energizing and uplifting. And the studies of mantra chanting that we discussed in Chapter Three show important physiological benefits. Often a spontaneous chant will rise up after my Yoga and meditation practice in the morning, or in the sauna or whirlpool. I find I have more energy to climb the Catalina foothills in Tucson on my bike when I am chanting. Chanting keeps me awake and alert when I am driving, particularly on long trips. I usually keep a CD in my car of my favorite chants and sing along. Not only do I feel more energy, but also my heart feels more open to a deepening connection to the divine.

Prayer, in whatever form it takes and to whatever deity or higher power within, can not only lift the heart from the darkness of depression but may actually help others in their recovery from illness. Physician Larry Dossey, author of *Healing Words* and *Prayer Is Good Medicine*, suggests that the intercessory prayer studies that have been done show the "nonlocal" nature of consciousness—which is what the Yogis have been saying for thousands of years. Yogis have verified the vast nature of mind in their own experiences on the mat, when small self dissolves into Self with a capital *S*. The subjective feeling is not describable in words. There is a sense of connection to all that is: *Tat tvam asi*—You are that. If this subjective feeling represents a glimpse of infinite mind, then the prayer studies make sense. Intercessory prayers, in which patients who did not know they were being prayed for had a higher rate of recovery than those who were not being prayed for, work because in prayer we somehow enlist not only our own mind but the infinite mind of cosmic consciousness.

From Darkness to Light: Devotion to Guru

In the East, aligning oneself with a teacher has long been a venerated path toward realizing one's full potential. The word *guru* means "from darkness to light." Devotion to a guru, it is believed, can awaken the heart, moving the devotee from the darkness of ignorance (*avidya*) to the light of knowledge and love, which in many Yogic traditions are one and the same. A story is often told in Yogic traditions: A farmer is desperate for water, so he begins to dig a well. He digs a hole deep enough to peer inside—no water. So he digs another hole and another, and pretty soon his property is filled with shallow holes. His neighbor, meanwhile, has dug one hole deep beneath the surface of the earth. He has penetrated the water table and quenched his thirst. I have heard this tale repeated by several spiritual masters. It is told to illustrate the importance of aligning oneself with one spiritual tradition, following one teacher, maintaining, as it were, spiritual monogamy.

Sri Sri Ravi Shankar speaks of staying on one path after you have started it. "Don't go here and there always spiritual shopping. What you heard from the Guru, the master, takes a little while to become reality for you and become part of your life. It's like planting a seed. Having sown, then it becomes a plant and starts bearing fruit. In between, if you start sowing other seeds there or pulling the seedling out then nothing happens. It doesn't take root."[10]

Amrit Desai, the founder of Kripalu Yoga, used to say that if you have never heard a concert of classical music, it is much more difficult to learn to play it from sheet music. But if you meet a concert musician and fall in love with his music, you are more inspired to learn to play, too. "You have a yearning to know more about the music so that you can create that music for yourself." In the same way, a guru, even one who is unenlightened, as Desai himself claimed to be, models a way of being in the world. "To become like the guru," he once said, "helps you practice the teachings more easily than if you tried to practice the teachings without the model." When you practice the teachings given by the guru, your own *sat guru,* or true inner teacher, awakens. "The love you feel for the external guru is 'a vehicle for loving yourself.'"[11]

For *Bhakti* Yogis, surrender to the guru can be a metaphorical expression of the devotee's inner embrace of the Divine. For those devoted to a guru, there are three significant aspects that can promote emotional healing. First, from a Western psychological level, there is the opportunity for change through the relationship itself. The love of the guru, even a male guru, "is seen as the manifestation of the *Shakti* or the divine Mother," says Stephen Cope.[12] Much like the transference that develops in a therapeutic relationship between therapist and patient, the guru-disciple relationship can provide fertile ground for healing. The wounds we sustained in our earliest relationships with our primary caregivers have the potential to be healed in this new "mothering" relationship. The guru becomes a loving guide, providing a safe harbor in which the devotee may be able to work through the relationship difficulties he has had in the past.

Second, the loving connection to the guru can be the vehicle to loving the divinity within the self, the true inner *sat guru* (*sat* means truth). "Connection with the master," says David Burge, an Art of Living teacher and coauthor of a book about Sri Sri Ravi Shankar, "is the way that is old and new—the way home to yourself."[13] The love one feels for an idealized being such as a guru, who may or may not be enlightened, opens the heart to unconditional love, to the love of the divine. "Yogis developed an entire science of relationship," says Stephen Cope. "The relationship with a beloved teacher [guru] became the doorway to the most profound relationship with the beloved—God in her many guises and forms."[14]

And third, the idealized guru models an enlightened way of functioning in the world, toward which the disciple grows. Sitting with an enlightened master is like having a highly polished mirror held before us. First, we see ourselves more clearly. In the guru's expansive and radiant light, our pettiness or small intentions are reflected back to us. And in the guru's limitless compassion and unconditional love, we begin to see our potential.

The Guru path is, of course, mined with explosives that have the potential to damage as easily as heal. The first factor is the character and trustworthiness of the teacher. Countless devotees in a number of traditions have had their trust betrayed by teachers who did not live according to the principles they espoused. The second potential problem in the guru-disciple relationship is the same dilemma we face in every relationship where we give one person, be it minister, teacher, or therapist, authority: Does the unequal nature of such a relationship foster dependency? A wise teacher cautions his students to look to their own inner wisdom and not to him for answers to their life's questions. Time and again, such a teacher will shake off the power the student tries to give him. And yet those of us with codependent tendencies may too easily hand over our power to a charismatic teacher.

But devotion does not need to be channeled through a guru. The former Oxford don and passionate seeker Andrew Harvey was once on a guru path. He's a wonderful example of someone whose devotional nature found a channel to the divine through his guru, then developed a more direct means of access. Andrew, in my opinion, is a true Bhakti, Jnana, and Karma Yogi who is making a difference in the world. He met Mother Meera in 1978, and through the eighties his devotion to her manifested itself in books dedicated to or about her. However, he says that when he asked for her blessing of his loving commitment to his beloved Eryk, not only would she not give it but she asked him to dump

Eryk and change his sexual orientation for love of her. He was deeply wounded and set adrift, yet he found his own way, as a Bhakti Yogi, through loss and devastation, back to the divine, without the mediation of a guru. Through chanting, prayer, and adoration of the Divine Mother, Andrew has access to his wholeness, to his birthright as a human being born divine. In his writing and his teaching, he helps others access their own inherent and natural connection to the divine. No intermediary necessary.[15]

The Karma Path

> Let the beauty you love be what you do.
> There are hundreds of ways to kneel and kiss the ground.

—RUMI, from "Today, like every other day, we wake up empty"[16]

Out of loving devotion arises the desire to serve, so it is almost impossible to separate the Bhakti path from the Karma Yoga path. When we act without attachment to the outcome, we are practicing Karma Yoga, one of the routes to self-realization that Krishna outlines for Arjuna in the *Bhagavad Gita*. The Karma Yogi feels related to all living beings. "We are all one family," Swami Kripalu used to say. "I belong to you," participants in the Art of Living Course say to one another. When we practice random acts of kindness, when we volunteer at a homeless shelter or support a loved one through an illness, our spirits are lifted. "Action performed in the spirit of self-surrender has benign invisible effects," says Yoga scholar Georg Feuerstein. "It improves the quality of our being and makes us a source of uplift for others."[17] When we volunteer to sit with someone who is dying or read to a child, we are performing selfless service (*seva*). This kind of action is taken from a place of love, from a spirit of self-surrender, from a place without attachment to the rewards of the service you are providing. And you are the biggest beneficiary of your service to others, because it makes you feel good about yourself.

Selfless service is good practice for developing the capacity to love without expectations, without clinging and seeking to possess. This kind of love is the ultimate love, unconditional, perhaps even more healing for the one who loves than the one who is loved. This is truly what it means to feel connected, to feel your love expanding beyond the limits of your physical body.

Many Yogic traditions understand how selfless service opens the heart to love. If you have ever volunteered to read to preschoolers, tutored children who are having difficulty reading, visited the elderly in a nursing home, or simply spent time attending others in need, you will have some understanding of how the heart is opened by seva. In my own case, the class I lead as a volunteer, teaching Yoga to girls between twelve and seventeen detained in the Cape School, the juvenile detention center in Tucson, Arizona, makes me happier than anything else I do.

Adolescence is a hard time for girls, a time of uncertainty, confusion, and even self-loathing. Added to the normal and not-so-normal pressures on girls of that age, the girls at the Cape School already have labels attached that may follow them for life. For these girls, the bad things that have been done to them have been projected out, sometimes in violent self-abuse, sometimes toward others. I share a little about this experience to illustrate how what we do for others, in the spirit of self-surrender, lifts us, according to Feuerstein, "by our own bootstraps out of the morass of mental conditionings."[18]

"What's my name?" the girls ask me as they line up, hoping I will remember them from last week. I remember each one of them, of course, but not always their names, which are often, to this middle-aged, middle-class Anglo, unfamiliar and hard to pronounce. Guadalupe, Tanika, Mercedez, Brandy, Christalia, Belen—these are Hispanic names, Native American names, Anglo names, African American names. Together we move out onto the cement courtyard, where we set up our dusty vinyl-covered mats in a circle on the even dustier cement, under the fenced-in desert sky.

We begin with a check-in—their names followed by a word or two about how they're feeling. The girls say they feel "fat," "sad," "depressed," "confused." I explain to "sad and mad" Miranda, whose voice is a whisper and whose eyes gaze downward, that Yoga will bring balance into her emotional body as well as her physical body. I ask her to tell me how she feels when the class is over.

Some girls are slow to respond, and it takes a while to get around the circle. Already, I can see I have lost Miranda and Tanika to their own frightening states of mind. Others are cracking whispered jokes, lying down. I want to engage them in a practice that may change their lives, so I bring them to their hands and knees to roar out their frustrations in Lion Pose. I tell them to scare away all the demons—anyone who has hurt them—and they make fierce faces and stick out their tongues and yell until the guards come running, and everyone giggles, then they rest for a few moments in Child Pose, with their foreheads on their mats, their buttocks on their heels, and their arms alongside their bodies. With their permission—many of the girls have been touched in pleasurable and painful ways without their permission—I give them back presses. "That feels like what my mother used to do," says Chica. "Do me, do me, Missy, do me," Tanika cries out.

Out of Child Pose, their faces are softer and it is easier to lead them through warm-ups and asanas. There is no protocol in these classes. Nothing like the quiet listening and following of instruction in a middle-class Yoga studio. Despite my instructions to move slowly and to pay attention to the sensations in their bodies, it is not unusual for two or three girls to try to outdo each other. They will move too quickly into the pose, exaggerate the movements, and intentionally fall out of Triangle or another stable standing pose, just for the group's reaction.

But there are moments when they are truly engaged, when after practicing Mountain (*Tadasana*) or Warrior (*Virabhadrasana*), they stand with eyes closed, feeling their energy, feeling how much bigger they are than their physical bodies.

I don't ask them what they did to wind up here. Terrible things have happened to these girls. When they're released, they will likely return to environments where more terrible things will happen. They may follow their karmic blueprint, reacting in ways that do damage to themselves and others. But in the hour we spend together, I hope that the Yoga not only lifts their spirits—and yes, Miranda says she feels better after our session—but that it also shows them their true and authentic selves. From this place of wholeness, perhaps they can see an alternative to the violence that has thus far characterized their lives. I remind them again and again that the energy they feel as they practice is who they really are—powerful, beautiful, radiant, and loving. For a moment, standing tall with their eyes closed and their palms open to receive, I think they believe me.

By the end of Yoga class, each is resting in Corpse Pose on her back (*shavasana*)—most with eyes closed. How precious and innocent they are, how trusting and vulnerable. Once, during their relaxation, as I was moving around the circle massaging their feet, I noticed a girl named Carmen with her eyes closed, whispering rapidly to herself. A psychotic episode? I wondered. Then I saw Gracia, the girl on the next mat, nod her head. As I knelt to massage Gracia's feet, I could hear Carmen's words: "Give your troubles to God," she was counseling Gracia. "He understands. He loves you. Your baby daughter loves you and knows you love her."

My heart breaks open at the end of nearly every class, just as it did that day, and I lead them in a final "Om," often with tears rolling down my face, feeling that this is the work I am meant to do. That here, in the presence of these pure but damaged spirits, is where my own karmic knots will finally unravel. Years of spiritual discipline could not open my heart the way the girls at the Cape School do every week. This is the effect of my selfless-service (seva)—my own heart lifting and opening.

And there are subtle changes in them, too, after the hour we spend together. In a preliminary study of the emotional effects of a single Kripalu Yoga class, participants reported increased feelings of happiness, peacefulness, and relaxation after class and less sadness, anger, and confusion. There was a major decrease in feelings of worry (52 percent) and a major increase in feelings of peacefulness (43 percent), suggesting that though difficult emotions may remain, the participants may be better able to cope with them after Yoga class.[19]

I wish I could tell you that the girls are empowered by their once-a-week practice and that their lives are dramatically changed. But the program is too informal and my time with them too short to know what the long-term effect of Yoga has been or will be in their lives. I can only tell you that working through their resistances to teach them Yoga each week is having a profound effect on me. Doing this nurturing work allows me to accept myself as I am—a flawed being who is dedicated to lifting the spirits of those around her, to helping them remember their wholeness.

Love and service lift the heart and dissipate the self-absorbed, obsessive thinking inherent in depression. It is impossible for me to be obsessing about my own problems after I've spent an hour with the girls at the Cape School. The service you do opens your heart, so that you feel more loving. And as you feel more loving, you naturally want to do more service. Love and service are the union of bhakti and karma Yoga. They nourish each other and they nourish you. And love and service may be the final step toward enlightenment. Service is the twelfth and final step in the recovery programs based on the Alcoholics Anonymous model. When the great nineteenth-century Bengali saint Ramakrishna was asked by an old woman how, after years of spiritual practice as a house-holder, she might finally reach enlightenment before she died, he asked her whom she loved more than anything or anyone else in the world. My precious granddaughter, she said. "Then go home and serve your grand-daughter," he told her. "That is your doorway to enlightenment."

True Community

> The purpose of
> every gathering is discovered:
>
> to recognize beauty and to love
> what's beautiful.
>
> —RUMI, from "Bowls of Food"[20]

If you live in a large enough town, there are gatherings of like-hearted people chanting to the divine, feeling their connection to the universe and each other in regular chanting events called *satsanga*, which means "contact with the real" or "in the company of truth." This can mean a community gathered to sit with a saint or a sage. For example, you may see a newspaper ad or a flyer for a satsanga with a visiting master teacher from India. But we also use the word "satsanga" to connote a gathering of like-hearted people in community. Finding your true community or satsanga is about finding a circle of friends with whom you can be utterly and completely yourself. Where the friendships and intimacies that develop are authentic. You don't have to chant to be part of a commu-nity. Your community may be through your church, your temple, your twelve-step meeting, or your Full Moon Circle. The research referred to above also takes a look at the support of community in recovery from depression. For some, it is not the prayer that is most healing but simply being a part of a supportive community of faith.

Perhaps your satsanga is your Yoga class. Amid the sounds of the treadmills running over our heads and the balls bouncing off the walls of the court next door, my students and I in our 7:00 A.M. class at the Tucson Racquet Club are such a community. Over the years we've been practicing together, we've come to know a little bit about one another, checking in at the beginning of class, sharing our accomplishments and the changes in our lives. I call on eighty-four-year-old Dorothy at her condo if she doesn't show up, and give others a ring at home if they've gone missing for more than a class or two. Sometimes Cynthia brings her harmonium and leads a chant. Sometimes we offer the merits of our practice to a student who is ill and unable to attend. And sometimes we celebrate a class member with a group "Om" by placing them in the middle of the circle. These are not Yogis living in a spiritual community, and except for Cynthia, most of my students have never chanted before and would never, except for their love of Cynthia and of me, have tried it in their lives. They are on their way to work, to shop, a doubles tennis match at 9:00 A.M., or back home for their next cup of coffee. They have never heard the word "satsanga," but for many of my students, their 7:00 A.M. Yoga class has come to feel like their true community. It certainly feels that way for me. As I write this, I am spending nearly three months as scholar-in-residence at Kripalu Center in Lenox, Massachusetts. Though I am grateful to be here, spiritually nourished while I finish this book, and am enjoying teaching Yoga classes for the guests, I miss my true community, my 7:00 A.M. Yoga class in Tucson.

Yoga teacher MJ Bindu Deleckta creates true community in the classes she teaches in her Yoga studio on Martha's Vineyard, Massachusetts, and at the retreats she leads each winter in Mexico. She encourages her students to share before the beginning of class. "I consider myself the facilitator of this circle of beings, creating an atmosphere of spaciousness by simply asking, 'What's up today?' Then, watching their reactions, I may expand the inquiry to include 'What did you notice about your week that gave you the opportunity to practice something you became aware of about yourself in the last Yoga class?' We simply sit together, breathe, and allow the responses to flow out from the heart." MJ Bindu calls this the "Sacred Circle" of Yoga, and indeed, the space she clears in her class through the sharing process is sacred. Over time, students begin to develop enough trust to "speak their truth." This is what it takes to create true community.

Finding Your Teacher

If many of our depressions are the result of a failure in relationship with our earliest caregivers, if we didn't receive enough of what we needed—that holding and soothing container that a loving relationship provides—then the nurturing relationships we create for ourselves as adults are crucial to our recovery. The one-to-one relationship you create with your Yoga teacher or Yoga therapist can be a nurturing model for self-healing. This means that the *quality* of that relationship is vital. Ask the questions of your potential teacher and his students posed in Chapter One to determine if he is the kind of teacher who can create a "good enough" emotional container in his Yoga class whereby you may begin to heal.

While traveling across the country, I once took an Ashtanga Yoga class in a western city. The studio was beautiful—high ceilings and long, arched windows through which the angled evening sun cast warrior shadows across the hardwood floor. This was a busy studio, and classes were scheduled back-to-back. Within moments of entering the practice room, I stood side by side with other students at the top of a purple sticky mat, facing a line of unsmiling practitioners, our hands in prayer position, ready to begin. What astonished me was that not a word of welcome had been spoken before we began the opening prayer—not from teacher to students, nor even a friendly "hello" between classmates.

The class was fine. The instructor's directions were clear, her adjustments were helpful, and the class proceeded through the sequence of postures much like every other primary series class. Don't misunderstand me. What I am describing—the lack of interaction, lack of satsanga, lack of that container of acceptance so essential in a class that is cognizant of the emotional body as well as the physical body—can take place in any Yoga class, regardless of the style of practice. I have attended Ashtanga classes where the teacher's warmth and connection to his students were evident from the first greeting to the final "Om." Tom Gillette, for example, a former Kripalu teacher-trainer, who at one time taught the Ashtanga Primary Series and has since developed his own flow of postures that he teaches in his Rhode Island studio, taught Ashtanga from a place of heart-to-heart connection with his students. It's just the way Tom is, no matter what kind of Yoga he is teaching. He often began by asking students to lift their hearts, to smile into their hearts, to expand their hearts. The joy and energy he brought to his Ashtanga classes were infectious, and though his Primary Series was pretty much like everyone else's, his students left feeling filled and stretched, emotionally as well as physically.

If the instructor creates an environment for practice where compassion takes precedence over the compulsion to "get it right," then even a Bikram Yoga class, known for its adherence to the exact duplication of every posture, can feel like a community of like-hearted practitioners. What this means is that even more important than finding the right style of Yoga is finding a teacher with whom you feel comfortable. If you're suffering from depression, no matter what style of Yoga you are practicing, the container of self-acceptance the teacher creates for the class is essential.

Finding Your Style

So maybe you've heard about a wonderful teacher, but how do you know if the style of Yoga she is teaching is right for your body? First of all, if she's really a good teacher and this is a beginning class, go for it. Let yourself have the experience of a first-rate, caring teacher, no matter what style of Yoga she is teaching. Learn the basics of her approach, then as you become more familiar with the variations in Yoga styles— perhaps you've picked up a book by a teacher from a different lineage, or seen ads in a Yoga magazine for a variety of Yoga trainings—try a class in a different style. Keep an open mind as you go to your new teacher's class. You are only limiting your own experience if, in your mind, you are constantly making comparisons, constantly thinking, "Well, *my* teacher would never do that!"

In Chapter Five, we talked about three different approaches: First we looked at Iyengar Yoga, which begins with an emphasis on willful practice (tapas), working primarily with the physical body to start. We also looked at Viniyoga, a style of Yoga that begins with an emphasis on self-study (svadhayaya). Finally, we looked at Kripalu Yoga, which starts you off with an exploration of all three aspects of practice—willful practice and self-study with surrender (Ishvara-pranidhana). And as we saw in Chapter Five, the three approaches, when you have practiced long enough, can bring you to that depression-free state of union that is Yoga. In other words, no matter what doorway you walk through, you eventually find yourself in the same place, seated in the center of the lotus.

Unless you're practicing an athletic and active form of Yoga like Ashtanga or Bikram for more than an hour every day, Yoga isn't a substitute for your exercise routine. I continue to work out with weights a couple of times a week and to ride a bike. I look to my Yoga practice not for aerobic exercise, but to release the impurities in my system so that I have more energy, think more clearly, and am not depressed. As I described my experience on the mat in Chapter Five, I also look to my practice to free me of the obstacles that keep me from remembering my wholeness. Any style of Yoga has the capacity to do this, to give you access to the feeling of energy that breaks the boundaries of your physical body.

But let's take a look at the styles of practice you're likely to find. If your teacher advertises herself as a "Hatha" Yoga instructor, it might be useful to probe a little deeper, because, as we've already learned, "Hatha" means physical force, and therefore all physical aspects of Yoga practice are considered Hatha Yoga. You might ask her if she identifies with any one particular tradition. If she's not certified or aligned with any tradition, it could be that she's studied with teachers from a number of traditions and has many years of experience teaching Yoga. Ask her who her primary teachers have been and in what style. You may not want to take your first Yoga class from someone who has learned her routine from a wide selection of videos or who has simply attended a series of Yoga classes at the YMCA. Your teacher doesn't have to be certified in a particular tradition to be qualified to teach, but ask her about her own learning and teaching experience before you sign up.

Since the mid-nineties the Yoga Alliance has been registering teachers. To be registered with the Yoga Alliance, an applicant must demonstrate minimum teaching standards that include knowledge of Yoga asana and philosophy. Until the end of 2002, even teachers who had not been trained and certified in a particular lineage were able to demonstrate that their training and studies with individual teachers qualified them to be registered with the Yoga Alliance. Ask your potential teacher if he is registered with the Yoga Alliance. It's an indication that he has met certain standards of training, but it is not the only criterion. There are many senior teachers who, on principle, wish not to be registered. They see Yoga as a transmission between teacher and student and may feel that any certification or registration process interferes with that relationship, setting up some kind of a hierarchy of "better than" and "best." Victor van Kooten and Angela Farmer have quietly crusaded against the certification process since B.K.S. Iyengar initiated it in his trainings in the seventies. Yet they are both master teachers from whom you may learn a lot about your own authentic expression of a pose.

Now let's take a look at some of the schools of Hatha Yoga. We discussed Iyengar Yoga, Viniyoga, and Kripalu Yoga in Chapter Five, but they are by no means the only or even the best-known schools. There are hundreds of traditions of Yoga, so please don't be concerned if your teacher doesn't come from one of the styles of practice I mention here. More important than the style are the attributes of the teacher, which we discussed in Chapter Five.

Bikram Yoga may be a good detoxing practice for your body. The class is held in a room heated to about 104 degrees, so the body sweats profusely in the twenty-six-posture, each-done-twice sequence. This sequence was designed by Bikram Choudry, a Yoga "champ" from India who, from his Los Angeles studio, teaches Yoga to the stars. After a class, Bikram practitioners, and I have been one of them, often feel as though the body has been cleansed. Certainly the lymphatic system, as in other forms of Yoga where postures are held for a specified time then released, is cleansed. The practice systematically warms and stretches muscles, ligaments, and tendons in the order in which Bikram feels they should be stretched. Many of the poses stimulate the glands, releasing hormones and therefore hormone production, so there is often a feel-good response.

Students are commanded, sometimes barked at, to maintain their alignment. In a Bikram class, the sequence is the same every time, so the mind is freed from the worry of what to do next and how to do it.

There's a comfort in the familiarity of the routine. This may be appealing to someone suffering from an anxiety-based depression or obsessive-compulsive disorder (OCD). The practice is vigorous and somewhat like a workout, which may work well to engage an anxiety-prone person, who may feel understimulated in a slower class. The practice is dynamic throughout, to be practiced with the eyes open. The final relaxation in Corpse Pose (Shavasana), the only time students may close their eyes, is usually not longer than a minute or two. Often students leave the class feeling more energized than relaxed.

The caution here is to find a teacher who is bigger than the limits of the practice, who can bring warmth and acceptance and humor into the practice room, and who understands that flexibility in the emotional body is as important as it is in the physical body. There are wonderful Bikram teachers who can create that kind of container for the class. On the other hand, you may wish to avoid a teacher whose basic personality seems aligned with the drill-sergeant aspects of being a Bikram teacher. Choose wisely.

Any of the Vinyasa Yoga flows, which include Ashtanga Yoga as taught by Pattabhi Jois, student of Krishnamacharya, or flows inspired by Ashtanga Yoga like Power Yoga, as taught by Beryl Bender Birch, or Jivamukti Yoga as taught by Sharon Gannon and David Life and White Lotus as taught by Tracey Rich and Ganga White, can be especially stimulating and perhaps a good choice of practice for someone who is fit and energetic, with a tendency toward anxiety-based depression. The flow begins vigorously, heating the body with sun salutations. Practitioners literally jump in and out of poses. After moving you through an exact sequence of postures, the practice usually concludes with a short, calming meditation and relaxation.

Longtime Yoga practitioner and teacher John Friend, who was a student of both Pattabhi Jois and B.K.S. Iyengar, has developed Anusara Yoga, a more heart-centered practice than the ones in which he was trained. Anusara literally means "to step into the current of Divine Will," or "flowing with grace." The emphasis in Anusara Yoga is on both outer and inner body alignment.

Ananda Yoga is among the traditions with a gentler, more meditative approach that includes an awareness of the importance of balancing the emotional body through practice. In the tradition of Paramahansa Yogananda, Ananda Yoga uses affirmations along with asana and pranayama to awaken, experience, and begin to control the subtle energies within. The intention of this practice is to use the awakened energies of the chakras to harmonize body, mind, and emotions, and above all to attune oneself with higher levels of awareness.

According to Swami Satchidananda, its founder, Integral Yoga is a synthesis of all the forms of Yoga. The Hatha aspect of an Integral practice includes asanas, pranayamas, and *kriyas* (cleansing processes), and mental concentration "to create a supple and relaxed body; increased vitality; radiant health; and help in curing physical illness."[21] The practice is designed to develop every aspect of the individual: physical, emotional, intellectual, and spiritual. Dr. Dean Ornish uses Integral Yoga in his groundbreaking work on reversing heart disease.

Yogi Bhajan is considered by his followers to be the *"Mahan Tantric,"* or highest living Yoga master in the world. In 1969, he brought his understanding of Kundalini Yoga to the West and since then has trained many teachers. A Kundalini class is quite active, with repetition of simple movements, rapid-breathing exercises, and active meditations that sometimes use mantra (tones or chants), mudra (hand movements or seals), breath, and visualization. The effect of a typical Kundalini class is usually a great surge of energy.

This practice has been helpful to many people suffering from dysthymia, but caution should be exercised when suffering from anxiety or bipolar disorder. The increased energy in the upper chakras, which often creates feelings of euphoria, may in certain cases trigger a manic episode. Within Kundalini Yoga there are practices that calm and soothe the energy; however, most Kundalini teachers spend more time raising the energy than calming it. If you are suffering from bipolar disorder, it is better to seek advice from a qualified teacher before entering a class. Most Kundalini teachers reflect the bright energy that is stimulated in their practice. It is especially important to talk to the teacher before beginning your practice to feel whether there's a fit, and if you're suffering from anxiety or bipolar disorder, that she has a thorough understanding of the exercises that will be most beneficial for you.

A Sivananda Yoga class will provide you with a full experience of pranayamas and classic asanas, followed by a relaxation. The practice was developed by Vishnu-Devananda and named for his teacher, Sivananda. In order to simplify the complex practices of Yoga, Swami

Vishnu-Devananda developed the five-point system that includes proper exercise (asana), proper breathing (pranayama), proper relaxation (shavasana), proper diet (vegetarianism), and positive thinking and meditation. Sivananda Yoga is based on the nondualist Advaita Vedanta philosophy, in which there is no reality but God and God is in every individual.

There are many other contemporary styles that have developed from the primary lineages. In Svaroopa Yoga, Rama Berch teaches a somewhat different approach to entering and holding a posture by working with the progressive alignment of the spine. Svaroopa, the term Patanjali uses in the *Yoga Sutras* to describe the essence of one's true nature, is a "consciousness-oriented Yoga that also promotes healing and transformation. Svaroopa is not an athletic endeavor, but a development of consciousness using the body as a tool."[22]

Practicing today are many fine senior teachers who've moved from their roots in Iyengar, Ashtanga, Sivananda, Kripalu, or other traditions to develop their own distinctive styles. Among them are Shiva Rea, Rama Jyoti Vernon, Rama Berch, John Friend, Tom Gillette, Ann Greene, Todd Norian, Dr. Jeff Migdow, Baron Baptiste, Rodney Yee, Ana Forrest, Angela Farmer, Victor Van Kooten, Sharon Gannon, David Life, and many others. Usually, in the development of their practices, these teachers have added a dimension of Western psychological awareness to the teachings they received from their Indian masters. And yet they are not deviating at all from the essence of Yoga as outlined in the *Yoga Sutras*, which set forth guidelines for developing the body, the emotions, and the intellect so that they function in harmony with one another.

When to Practice?

People who are depressed suffer most in the early hours of the morning. This is when suicides are most likely to occur.[23] So it is good therapy to practice in the morning, even if you have to drag yourself out of bed to do so. Take a shower to wake yourself up (Yogi Bhajan suggests that Kundalini Yogis begin with a cold shower every morning), then head for your Yoga class or roll out your mat in your living room, put in a videotape or audiotape if you need motivation, and begin a practice. If you get the prana flowing first thing in the morning, if you stretch and breathe in

ways that calm and energize your mind, chances are you won't carry your
depression with you through your day.

Finally

Just as when I say good-bye to my Tucson students to go off to teach
somewhere else, I feel a pang of sorrow now, ending this book and saying good-bye to you. Though if I saw you on the street I wouldn't recognize you (and this troubles me), I feel we've shared an experience. We've
explored the path of Yoga together, we've explored your symptoms
together, and we've considered Yogic techniques that work best for you.
In our journey through this book, we've created a kind of relationship. I
hope it's one that has inspired you to begin or to deepen your own practice, finding new ways to heal from your depression. And I hope that we
can meet in person in a workshop soon. I want our recognition of each
other to be mutual. I want to say, "Ah, there you are, the man from
Cincinnati who . . ." or "the woman from Chicago who . . ." I want us
to be able to look into each other's eyes and recognize each other's
magnificence!

I will close with a reminder and a wish. First, *please* practice every
day in some way. You don't take your antidepressant three times a week.
Like medication, for Yoga to be effective, you need a daily dose.

And finally: May your practice help free you from the obstacles that
keep you from remembering your wholeness!

Jai Bhagwan and *Namaste*
I bow to the divine within you.

yoga experience

1. Karma Yoga: Random Act of Kindness

This is a simple practice, and if you do it every day, you will be inviting loving kindness into your life. Find an opportunity to offer assistance to someone. Opportunities are everywhere. Perhaps as you're brushing the snow from your windshield, you clean off the windshield of the car beside you. Or you might give up your seat in the subway. Or let the person behind you in line check out his groceries first. Or buy a book you love for a friend. No reason. Just give someone else a moment of pleasure. You will feel good about yourself.

2. Jnana Yoga: *The Yoga Sutras*

Read one of Patanjali's *Yoga Sutras* before and after your morning practice and ask for guidance about how it might apply to your own life. Here's an example; this is the second sutra in Chapter One:

> *Yogas-citta-vrtti-nirodhah.*
> Yoga is the cessation of identifying with the fluctuations of consciousness.[24]

You might recite this sutra in Sanskrit or English several times, then ask yourself with what thoughts or feelings you are identifying. Each time you cling to a thought or a feeling or a sensation, you are creating suffering for yourself in the form of separation. As you practice Yoga, you begin to cultivate the Witness, a consciousness that allows you to observe your passing thoughts and feelings without identifying with them. For example, you may observe that you feel depressed today. This awareness is very different from telling yourself that you *are* depressed. When you see your depressed mood from the place of the Witness, you recognize that it is a fluctuating state, that it will change, that it is not who you really are.

3. Bhakti Yoga: Practice Prayer

The next time you practice, ask that there be no obstacles, no walls between you and the divine. Or use the following prayer:

Sadhana (Practice) Prayer

Here I am! Your vessel,
Ready to be filled with your breath.
Let me feel you in every sensation.
Let me touch you as my fingertips touch each other.
Let me see you in the light behind my eyes.
Let me hear you in the sound of my breath.
Let the river of your love flow through me.
Let there be no separation!
No longer an "us."
Only the one true Self.
I am.
Tat tvam asi—*I am that.*

Epigraph

1. Swami Kripalu as quoted by Aruni Nan Futuronsky, "Kripalu Yoga Off the Mat: Choosing to Be Present," *Kripalu Yoga Association Yoga Bulletin,* Vol. 12, 2 (2003), p. 11.

Chapter One: Empty Pockets

1. Coleman Barks, trans., "The Pattern Improves," *The Soul of Rumi: A New Collection of Ecstatic Poems* (New York: HarperSanFrancisco, 2001), p. 31.

2. Maryanna Eckberg, Ph.D., "Shock Trauma: Case Study of a Survivor of Political Torture," *The Body in Psychotherapy*. Don Hanlon Johnson and Ian J. Grand, eds. (Berkeley, California: North Atlantic Books, 1998), p. 18.

3. Mark Epstein, M.D., *Thoughts Without a Thinker: Psychotherapy from a Buddhist Perspective* (New York: Basic Books, 1995), p. 30.

4. Ibid., p. 38.

5. *McMan's Depression and Bipolar Weekly* 3, #48 & #44. (2001), www.jmcmanamy@snet.net.

6. Peter D. Kramer, *Listening to Prozac* (New York: Penguin Books, 1993), pp. 119–121.

7. Stephen Cope, *Yoga and the Quest for the True Self* (New York: Bantam, 1999), p. 39.

8. For a more thorough discussion of the *kleshas* from a psychological perspective, see Stephen Cope's *Yoga and the Quest for the True Self* (New York: Bantam, 1999), pp. 63–65.

Chapter Two: A House on Fire—The Ways We Suffer

1. Sri Sri Ravi Shankar, "The Six Distortions of Love," *Wisdom for the New Millenium* (Santa Barbara, California: Art of Living Foundation, 1999), p. 171.

2. Anne Cushman, "Into the Heart of Sorrow," *Yoga Journal* (March/April, 2001).

3. Alexander Lowen, M.D., "The Energy Dynamics of Depression: Healing Depression Through Bodywork," *Sacred Sorrows,* John E. Nelson and Andrea Nelson, editors. (New York: A Jeremy P. Tarcher/Putnam Book), p. 106.

4. Noah Sadek, M.D., Charles Nemeroff, M.D., Ph.D., "Update on the Neurobiology of Depression" (2001), www.medscape.com.

5. Suzanne Ironbiter, "The Goddess's Promise," *Devi* (Stamford, CT: Yuganta Press, 1987), p. 33.

6. This sequence can be found in *Yoga: The Path to Holistic Health* by B.K.S. Iyengar (London: Dorling Kindersley, 2001)

7. Kirsten Trabbic Michaels, M.A., "Yoga Therapy and Post-Traumatic Stress Disorder," *Yoga Studies* (Yoga Research and Education Center [YREC], 2002).

8. Mercedes A. McCormick, Ph.D., RYT, "Yoga Therapy: Road to Resiliency— Helping People Heal in the Wake of Terrorist Attacks," *Yoga Studies* (Yoga Research and Education Center [YREC], 2002).

9. William Styron, *Darkness Visible: A Memoir of Madness* (New York: Vintage Books, 1990), p. 19.

10. Thomas Lewis, M.D., Fari Amini, M.D., Richard Lannon, M.D., *A General Theory of Love* (New York: Random House, 2000), p. 70.

11. Peter D. Kramer, M.D., *Listening to Prozac* (New York: Penguin Books, 1993, 1997), pp. 212–215.

12. Sadek and Nemeroff, ibid.

13. Joshua Logan, *Josh: My Up and Down, In and Out Life* (New York: Delacorte Press, 1976), p. 147.

14. Kay Redfield Jamison, *Touched with Fire: Manic Depressive Illness and the Artistic Temperament* (New York: Simon & Schuster, 1993), p. 16.

15. Leonard Woolf, *Beginning Again: An Autobiography of the Years 1911–1918* (New York: Harcourt, 1964), pp. 172–174.

16. Joyce Carol Oates, *Solstice* (New York: E. P. Dutton, 1985), pp. 106–107.

17. Kay Redfield Jamison, ibid., p. 192.

18. Anne Sexton, "The Sickness Unto Death," *That Awful Rowing Toward God* (Boston: Houghton Mifflin Company, 1975), p. 40.

19. Styron, p. 17.

20. Thomas Moore, *Care of the Soul* (New York: HarperCollins, 1992), p. 140.

21. Bernadette Roberts, *The Experience of No-Self* (New York: State University of New York Press, 1993), p. 67.

22. Moore, p. 146.

23. Tim Farrington, "Hell of Mercy," *The Sun* (March, 2001), p. 29.

24. Swami Venkatesananda, *Enlightened Living* (Sebastopol, CA: Anahata Press, 1998), No. II, p. 44.

25. Gary Kraftsow, *Yoga for Wellness: Healing with the Timeless Teachings of Viniyoga* (New York: Penguin Putnam, 1999), p. 319.

Chapter Three: Why Yoga Works

1. Mirabai, "A Hundred Objects Close By," trans. Daniel Ladinsky, *Love Poems from God: Twelve Sacred Voices from the East and West* (New York: Penguin Compass, 2002), p. 245.

2. Erik Hoffman, Ph.D., "Mapping the Brain's Activity after Kriya Yoga," www.scan-Yoga.org.

3. G. Brainard, V. Pratap, C. Reed, B. Levitt, J. Hanifin, "Plasma Cortisol Reduction in Healthy Volunteers Following a Single Yoga Session of Yoga Practices," *Yoga Research Society Newletter* (Philadelphia, PA: Neurology, Jefferson Med. Col., 1997), No. 18.

4. Lisa Slède, M.A., and Rachel Pomerantz, "Yoga and Psychotherapy: A Review of the Literature," *International Journal of Yoga Therapy* (Santa Rosa, California: Yoga Research and Education Center, 2001), No. 11, p. 64. The authors review an article by B. Auriol in *Psychothérapies Psychosomatic,* 1972, 20:162–168.

5. Sat Bir S. Khalsa, Ph.D., "Treating Depression: A Review of the Scientific Evidence," *Aquarian Times,* Winter 2001.

6. S. Telles, R. Nagarathna, H. R. Nagendra, T. Desiraju, "Physiological Changes in Sports Teachers Following Three Months of Training in Yoga," *Indian Journal of Medical Science* (1993), Oct. 47(10):235–238.

7. John J. Austin, Ph.D., Shauna L. Shapiro, M.A., Roberta A. Lee, M.D., and Dean H. Shapiro, Jr., Ph.D., "The Construct of Control in Mind-Body Medicine: Implications for Health Care," *Alternative Therapies* (1999), Vol. 5, No. 2.

8. Dharma Singh Khalsa, M.D., *Meditation as Medicine: Activate the Power of Your Natural Healing Force* (New York: Pocket Books, 2001), p. 111.

9. Mehmet C. Oz, M.D., quoted by Alison Rose Levy, "Om Is Where the Heart Is," *Yoga Journal,* July/August 2002.

10. Dharma Singh Khalsa, M.D., Ibid., p. 115. For a fascinating in-depth look at *Naad Yoga,* the Yoga of sound, from a physiological as well as a spiritual perspective, see "Chapter Six—Mantra: The Tides and Rhythms of the Universe."

11. J. D. Teasdale, R. V. Segal, J. M. G. Williams, V. A. Ridgeway, J. M. Soulsby, M. A. Lau, "Prevention of Relapse/Recurrance in Major Depression by Mindfulness-Based Cognitive Therapy," *Journal of Counseling and Clinical Psychology 2000,* Vol. 68, No. 4, p. 622.

12. Stephen Cope, *Yoga and the Quest for the True Self* (New York: Bantam, 1999), pp. 127–135.

13. Lisa Slède, M.A., Rachel Pomerantz, ibid., p. 64. The authors review an article by J.R.M. Goyeche, "Yoga as Therapy in Psychosomatic Medicine," *Psychotherapy and Psychosomatics,* 1977, 31:373–381.

14. S. Telles, V. Ramaprabhu, S. K. Reddy, "Effect of Yoga Training on Maze Learning," *Indian Journal of Physiological Pharmacology* (April 2000), 44(2):197–201.

15. N. K. Manjunath, S. Telles, "Factors Influencing Changes in Tweezer Dexterity Scores Following Yoga Training," *Indian Journal of Physiological Pharmacology* (1999 April), 43(2):225–229.

16. P. Raghuraj, S. Telles, "Muscle Power, Dexterity Skill and Visual Perception in Community Home Girls Trained in Yoga or Sports and in Regular School Girls," *Indian Journal of Physiological Pharmacology* (1997 Oct), 41(4):409–415.

17. Lisa Slède, M.A., Rachel Pomerantz, ibid., p. 69. The authors review an article by J. C. Smith, "Meditation as Psychotherapy: A Review of the Literature," *Psychological Bulletin,* 1975, 82(4):558–564.

18. Ibid., p. 67. The authors review an article by D. S. Shannahoff-Khalsa, "Clinical Case Report: Efficacy of Yogic Techniques in the Treatment of Obsessive-Compulsive Disorders," *International Journal of Neuroscience,* 1996, 85:1–17.

19. Ibid., p. 67. The authors review an article by E. Leskowitz, "Seasonal Affective Disorder and the Yoga Paradigm: A Reconsideration of the Role of the Pineal Gland," *Medical Hypotheses,* 1990, 33(3):155–158.

20. For a clear description of Downward-Facing Dog Pose, see *The Woman's Book of Yoga and Health* by Linda Sparrowe with Yoga sequences by Patricia Walden (Boston: Shambhala, 2002), p. 46.

21. For a clear description of Headstand, see *The Woman's Book of Yoga and Health* by Linda Sparrowe with Yoga sequences by Patricia Walden (Boston: Shambhala, 2002), p. 16-17.

22. There is some controvery about whether full Shoulderstand is safe. Some physiologists believe it can compress the cervical vertebrae. It is especially difficult for large bodies. Half-Shoulderstand is a safer alternative and has many of the same benefits. For a clear and safe description of Half-Shoulderstand, see *Kripalu Yoga: A Guide to Practice On and Off the Mat* by Richard Faulds and the Senior Teaching Staff at Kripalu Center for Yoga and Health (New York: Bantam Books, 2004).

23. Roger Cole, Ph.D., "Questions and Answers," *Yoga Studies Newsletter,* Yoga Research and Education Center (May–August, 2002).

24. John Kepner, "Yoga Therapy and Complementary and Alternative Medicine Policy," *Yoga Studies Newsletter,* Yoga Research and Education Center, (May–August, 2002).

25. Mukunda Stiles, "The Joint-Freeing Series: Pavanmuktasana," *Structural Yoga Therapy* (York Beach, Maine: Samuel Weiser, Inc., 2000), pp. 121–133.

26. Richard Faulds, *Kripalu Yoga: A Guide to Practice On and Off the Mat* (New York: Bantam Books, 2004).

Chapter Four: Fertilizing the Ground—The Healing Principles of Yoga

1. T.K.V. Desikachar, *The Heart of Yoga: Developing a Personal Practice* (Rochester, Vermont: Inner Traditions International, 1995), p. 6.

2. Swami Prabhavananda, Christopher Isherwood, "Intoduction to Shankara's Philosophy," *Shankara's Crest-Jewel of Discrimination: Timeless Teachings on Nonduality* (Hollywood, California: Vedanta Press, 3rd ed., 1978), p. 18.

3. Peter Singer, *How Are We to Live? Ethics in an Age of Self-Interest* (New York: Prometheus Books, 1995), p. 29.

4. Ibid., p. 32.

5. Ibid., p. 30.

6. Kohlberg, L., "Stage and Sequence: The Cognitive-Developmental Approach to Socialization," *Handbook of Socialization: Theory and Research*, D. Goslin, ed. (Chicago: Rand McNally, 1969).

7. Dennis L. Krebs, "The Evolution of Moral Dispositions in the Human Species," Annals of the New York Academy of Sciences (2000), 907:132–148.

8. Marshall Govindan, *Kriya Yoga Sutras of Patanjali and the Siddhas: Translation, Commentary and Practice* (Quebec, Canada: Kriya Yoga Publications, 2000), p. 94.

9. Georg Feuerstein, Ph.D., *The Yoga Tradition: Its History, Literature, Philosophy and Practice* (Prescott, Arizona: Hohm Press, 1998), p. 326.

10. Sri Sri Ravi Shankar, "The Eight Limbs of Yoga," *The Yoga Sutras of Patanjali: A Commentary by Sri Sri Ravi Shankar*, tape ten of a ten-part series (The Art of Living Foundation, 1995).

11. Feuerstein, p. 327.

12. Govindan, II.33, p. 99.

13. Lisa Powers, "Yoga for Emotional Healing" (videotape) Clarity Sound & Light, 2000.

14. Ibid.

15. Ibid.

16. Ibid.

17. Sri Sri Ravi Shankar, "Healing with Consciousness," *Wisdom for the New Millennium* (Santa Barbara, California: Art of Living Foundation, 1999), p. 54.

18. Victor Van Kooten as quoted by Amy Weintraub, "Sun, Surf & Savasana in the Yucatan," *Yoga Journal* (November/December, 2000), p. 21.

19. Julia Mines, "Words to Develop a Healthy Body Image," *Kripalu Yoga Teacher Association Yoga Bulletin*, Winter 98, vol. 7, issue 4, p. 11

Chapter Five: Lotus of Many Petals—The Ways We Practice

1. Jaladhin Rumi, "The Guest House," trans. Coleman Barks, *The Essential Rumi* (New York: HarperSanFrancisco, 1995), p. 109.

2. B.K.S. Iyengar, *Yoga: The Path to Holistic Health* (London: Dorling Kindersley, 2001), p. 13.

3. Ibid., p. 168.

4. Robert Perkins, "Journey in Yama-Yama Land," *How We Live Our Yoga*, Valerie Jeremijenko, ed. (Boston: Beacon Press, 2001), p. 114.

5. Ibid., p. 116.

6. For a description of Vipariti Karani, see *Yoga: The Path to Holistic Health* by B.K.S. Iyengar (London: Dorling Kindersley, 2001), p. 216.

7. For a description of Supta Virasana, see *Yoga: The Path to Holistic Health* by B.K.S. Iyengar (London: Dorling Kindersley, 2001), p. 146.

8. For a description of Supta Baddhakonasana, see *Yoga: The Path to Holistic Health* by B.K.S. Iyengar (London: Dorling Kindersley, 2001), p. 226.

9. For a description of Setu Bandhasana, see the Yoga Experience in Chapter Nine.

10. Gary Kraftsow as quoted by Amy Weintraub, "The Natural Prozac," *Yoga Journal* (Nov.–Dec., 1999), p. 134.

Chapter Six: Fire in the Belly—Managing with Yogic Breathing

1. Danna Faulds, "Breath," *Go In and In* (Kearney, Nebraska: Morris Publishing, 2002), p. 4.

2. André van Lysebeth, *Pranayama: The Yoga of Breathing* (London: Unwin Hyman Limited, 1979), p. 3.

3. Kurt Keutzer, "Kundalini: Frequently Asked Questions," http://www-cad.eecs.berkeley.edu/-keutzer/kundalini/kundalini-faq.html.

4. The Inner Quest Intensive is a "life-changing" program at Kripalu Center that challenges the emotional body. Participants spend 15 hours a day "in focused activities structured to produce optimal exploration and change." *Kripalu Program Guide* (winter/spring 2002) p. 70.

5. Donna Farhi, *The Breathing Book* (New York: Henry Holt and Company, 1996), p. 53.

6. Alan Hymes, M.D., "Respiration and the Chest: The Mechanics of Breathing," *Science of Breath: A Practical Guide* (Honesdale, Pennsylvania: The Himalayan Institute Press, 1979, 1988), p. 37.

7. Alexander Lowen, M.D., *Depression and the Body* (New York: Penguin Putnam, 1972), p. 85.

8. Ibid., p. 92.

9. Farhi, p. 50.

10. S. Telles, R. Nagarathna, H. R. Nagendra. "Physiological Measures of Right Nostril Breathing," *Journal of Alternative Complementary Medicine* (winter 1996), 2(4): 479–484.

11. David Coulter, Ph.D., "The Physiology of *Bhastrika*," *Yoga International*, www.yogainternational.com.

12. S. Telles, T. Desiraju, "Oxygen Consumption during Pranayamic Type of Very Slow-Rate Breathing," *Indian Journal of Medical Research* (October 1991), 94: 357–363.

Chapter Seven: Art of Living—Breathing That Heals

1. Rainer Maria Rilke, "*I'm so alone in the world*," *Rilke's Book of Hours: Love Poems to God,* trans. by Anita Barrows and Joanna Macy. (New York: Riverhead Books, 1996), p. 59.

2. Numerous abstracts and scientific papers in "Science of Breath," International Symposium on *Sudarshan Kriya, Pranayam* & Consciousness (March 2 and 3, 2002), AIIMS, New Delhi, India.

3. Verna Suarez, M.S., M.F.T., "Anxiety Study at Lance Alternative Program," *Science of Breath*, International Symposium on *Sudharshan Kriya, Pranayam* & Consciousness, March 2002, AIIMS, New Delhi, India.

4. Richard P. Brown, M.D., Patricia L. Gerbag, M.D., "Yogic Breathing and Meditation: When the Thalamus Quiets the Cortex and Rouses the Limbic System" (March 2002), unpublished.

5. David Burge, Gary Bouchele, *Sri Sri Ravi Shankar: The Way of Grace* (Santa Barbara, California: Art of Living Foundation, 1996), p.10.

6. Ibid.

7. Roy King, M.D., Ph.D., Ann Brownstone, M.S., O.T.R., "Neurophysiology of Yoga Meditation," *International Journal of Yoga Therapy* (1999), No. 9, p. 12.

8. Dharma Singh Khalsa, *Meditation as Medicine* (New York: Pocket Books, 2001), p. 105.

9. Kalpana Jain, "Pranayam Has Scientific Basis, Says US Expert," *The Times of India Online,* (March 3, 2002), www.timesofindia.com.

10. Interview by Michael Fischman, "Discovering the Yoga of Breath: A Conversation with Sri Sri Ravi Shankar" (Santa Barbara, California: Art of Living Foundation, 2000).

11. Burge and Boucherle, p. 6.

Chapter Eight: Meditate to Mediate

1. *Shankara's Crest Jewel of Discrimination: Timeless Teachings on Nonduality,* trans. Swami Prabhavananda and Christopher Isherwood (Hollywood, California: Vedanta Press, 3rd edition, 1978), pp. 92, 126.

2. Jane Hirshfield, "The Door," *The October Palace* (New York: Harper-Perennial, 1994), p. 40.

3. Mark Epstein, M.D., *Going to Pieces Without Falling Apart: A Buddhist Perspective on Wholeness* (New York: Broadway Books, 1998), p. 17.

4. Ibid.

5. John Tarrant, *The Light Inside the Dark* (New York: HarperCollins, 1998), p. 222.

6. Epstein, p. 6.

7. Richard Restak, M.D., *The Brain* (New York: Bantam, 1984), p. 118.

8. H. O. Landolt, J. C. Gillin, "Sleep Abnormalities During Abstinence in Alcohol-Dependent Patients: Aetiology and Management," *Central Nervous System Drugs* (2001), 15(5):413–425.

9. Epstein, p. 47.

10. Ibid.

11. Ibid., p. 10.

12. Daniel Goleman, "Finding Happiness: Cajole Your Brain to Lean to the Left," *New York Times* (February 4, 2003).

13. Ibid.

14. Linda Knittel, "House of Healing," *Yoga Journal* (December, 2002), p. 33.

15. Phillip Moffit, "Selfless Gratitude," *Yoga Journal* (July/August, 2002), p. 61.

16. Ibid., p. 62.

17. Roy King, M.D, Ph.D., and Ann Brownstone, M.S., O.T.R., "Neurophysiology of Yoga Meditation," *International Journal of Yoga Therapy*, (1999) No. 9, p. 14.

18. Sharon Salzberg, *Lovingkindness: The Revolutionary Art of Happiness* (Boston: Shambhala, 1995), p. 116.

19. For a more traditional Karuna practice, a beautiful essay on compassion, and other healing meditations, see Sharon Salzberg's *Lovingkindness: The Revolutionary Art of Happiness* (Boston: Shambhala, 1995).

Chapter Nine: Grief in the Tissues—Releasing Trauma

1. Danna Faulds, from "Go In and In," *Go In and In* (Kearney, Nebraska: Morris Publishing, 2002), p. 2.

2. Somatic psychotherapists practice a body-oriented psychotherapy, often incorporating movement, body-awareness exercises, and imaginative visualizations. For a thorough discussion of various somatic psychotherapeutic treatment modalities, see the excellent series of anthologies edited by Don Hanlon Johnson and Ian J. Grand, which include *Bone, Breath and Gesture, Groundworks,* and *The Body in Psychotherapy* (Berkeley: North Atlantic Press, 1998). Also see books in the field of bioenergetics by Alexander Lowen, including *Bioenergetics* (New York: Penguin, 1975) and *Depression and the Body* (New York: Penguin, 1972).

3. Richard Miller quoted by Amy Weintraub in "The Natural Prozac," *Yoga Journal* (Nov./Dec., 1999), p. 43.

4. Maryanna Eckberg, Ph.D., "Shock Trauma: Case Study of a Survivor of Political Torture," *The Body in Psychotherapy*, Don Hanlon Johnson and Ian J. Grand, eds. (California: North Atlantic Books, 1998), p. 19.

5. Thomas Lewis, M.D., Fari Amini, M.D., Richard Lannon, M.D., *A General Theory of Love* (New York: Random House, 2000), p. 177.

6. Eric Hoffman, Ph.D., "Mapping the Brain's Activity after Kriya Yoga," Scandinavian Yoga and Meditation School (1999), http://www.scand-yoga.org.

7. Michael Lee, *Phoenix Rising Yoga Therapy: A Bridge from Body to Soul* (Deerfield Beach, Florida: Health Communications, Inc., 1997), p. 17.

8. For more about the Trauma Bond, see Jan Hindman's *Just Before Dawn* (Oregon: Alexandria Associates, 1999).

9. Thomas Lewis, M.D., interviewed by Moira Gun on "Tech Nation"

(NPR broadcast on 12/15/2001). For a full discussion of the neurochemistry of our attractions, see *A General Theory of Love* by Thomas Lewis, M.D., Fari Amini, M.D., Richard Lannon, M.D. (New York: Random House, 2000).

10. Robert Karen, Ph.D., *Becoming Attached* (New York: Warner Books, 1994), pp. 234–235.

11. Mark Epstein, M.D., *Thoughts Without a Thinker* (New York: Basic Books, 1995), p. 52.

12. Lewis, Ibid.

13. Plough Pose (*Halasana*)—This inversion reverses the blood flow in the body, stimulates the endocrine system, and is a good posture to include toward the end of your practice. See *The Woman's Book of Yoga and Health* by Linda Sparrowe with Yoga sequences by Patricia Walden (Boston: Shambhala, 2002), p. 20.

14. Epstein (quoting Sigmund Freud), p. 17.

15. Epstein, p. 40.

16. Ibid.

17. Lee, pp. 13–14.

18. Lee, p. 14.

19. Epstein, p. 3.

20. Eckberg, p. 24.

21. This Yoga Experience is based on the Kripalu method of "Riding the Wave."

Chapter Ten: Yoga On and Off the Mat

1. Nelly Sachs, "Someone," *Women in Praise of the Sacred*, ed. Jane Hirshfield, trans. by Ruth and Matthew Mead (New York: HarperPerennial, 1994), p. 220.

2. Anon., "Ishvara-Gita: Song of the Divine," *Kurma-Purana*, quoted by Georg Feuerstein, Ph.D., *The Shambhala Encyclopedia of Yoga* (Boston, Massachusetts: Shambhala Publications, 1997), p. 132.

3. Swami Prabhavananda, Christopher Isherwood, *Shankara's Crest Jewel of Discrimination* (Hollywood, California: Vedanta Press, 1947, 1978), pp. 91–92.

4. Rainer Maria Rilke, "*I Believe in All*," trans. Anita Barrows, Joanna Macy, *Rilke's Book of Hours: Love Poems to God* (New York: Riverhead Books, 1996), p. 58.

5. Coleman Barks, trans. from "A Necessary Autumn Inside Each," *The Soul of Rumi: A New Collection of Ecstatic Poems* (New York: HarperSanFrancisco, 2001), p. 21.

6. Jane Lampman, "A Frontier of Medical Research: Prayer," *The Christian Science Monitor* (March 25, 1998).

7. Rabia of Basra, "In My Soul," trans. Daniel Ladinsky. *Love Poems from God: Twelve Sacred Voices from the East and West* (New York: Penguin Compass, 2002), p. 11.

8. Georg Feuerstein, Ph.D., *The Yoga Traditions: Its History and Literature* (Prescott, Arizona: Hohm Press, 1998), p. 48.

9. Stephen Mitchell, translator, *Bhagavad Gita* (New York: Harmony Books, 2000), 9(32–34), pp. 119–120.

10. Sri Sri Ravi Shankar, "Living All Possibilities in Life," *Wisdom for the New Millenium* (Santa Barbara, California: Art of Living Foundation, 1999), p. 185.

11. Yogi Amrit Desai, "Love Creates Oneness," audiotape, Kripalu Yoga Fellowship, 1988.

12. Stephen Cope, *Yoga and the Quest for the True Self* (New York: Bantam, 1999), p. 143.

13. David Burge, Gary Boucherle, *Sri Sri Ravi Shankar: The Way of Grace* (Santa Barbara, California: Art of Living Foundation, 1996), p. 3.

14. Cope, p. 143.

15. Andrew Harvey, *The Direct Path: Creating a Personal Journey to the Divine Using the World's Spiritual Traditions* (New York: Broadway Books, 2000).

16. Coleman Barks, trans. from "Today, like every other day, we wake up empty," *The Essential Rumi* (New York: HarperSanFrancisco, 1995), p. 36.

17. Georg Feuerstein, "The Desire for Liberation," *Yoga International* (July 2002), p. 28.

18. Ibid.

19. Amy Weintraub, MFA, RYT, in consultation with George Goldman, Ph.D., "Measurement of feelings before and after a one-hour Yoga class for females in juvenile detention" (June 2002), unpublished.

20. Coleman Barks, trans. from "Bowls of Food," p. 201.

21. Swami Satchidananda, *Integral Yoga Hatha* (New York: Henry Holt and Company, 1970), p. xv.

22. John Tunney, www.yogasite.com.

23. Richard Restak, M.D. *The Brain* (New York: Bantam, 1984), p. 118.

24. This translation of Sutra I.2 is taken from *Kriya Yoga Sutras of Patanjali and the Siddhas* by Marshall Govindan (Eastman, Quebec, Canada: Kriya Yoga Publications, 2000).

This is by no means an exhaustive list. These are simply the Yoga and psychological resources that I have found most inspiring and that have been helpful in my work with others still suffering from depression.

My Companions

The books in this first group are not necessarily about practice, and if they are, they place practice in a larger context of psychological, spiritual, and planetary well-being. Here are a few special books about Yoga, meditation, and spirituality that continue to inspire me.

Cope, Stephen. *Yoga and the Quest for the True Self.* New York: Bantam Books, 1999. A thorough and highly readable book that looks at the ancient tradition of Yoga in the context of contemporary psychological thinking.

Epstein, Mark, M.D. *Thoughts Without a Thinker.* New York: Basic Books, 1995. Written by a practicing Buddhist psychiatrist, this is a thoughtful consideration of Buddhist philosophy in the context of Western psychological thought.

Faulds, Richard, with the Senior Teaching Staff of Kripalu Center for Yoga and Health. *Kripalu Yoga: A Guide to Practice On and Off the Mat.* New York: Bantam Books, 2004. A beautiful theory and practice book that outlines the Three Stages of Kripalu Yoga—willful practice, self-observation with acceptance, and surrender—all that you need to recover from depression.

Jeremijenko, Valerie, editor. *How We Live Our Yoga: Personal Stories.* Boston: Beacon Press, 2001. Serious Yoga practitioners talk honestly about how Yoga has altered their lives. Included is a poignant essay by Robert Perkins about his recovery from depression.

Harvey, Andrew. *The Direct Path: Creating a Personal Journey to the Divine Using the World's Spiritual Traditions.* New York: Broadway Books, 2000. Part memoir, part book of spiritual practices by one of the world's most passionate thinkers and mystics, *The Direct Path* eschews gurus, priests, and spiritual masters to give readers a personal link to the divine.

Khalsa, Dharma Singh, M.D., and Stauth, Cameron. *Meditation as Medicine.* New York: Fireside, 2000. Written by a physician, this book includes theory and Kundalini meditation practices for various medical conditions, including depression.

Kraftsow, Gary. *Yoga for Wellness: Healing with the Timeless Principles of Viniyoga.* New York: Penguin Compass, 1999. A practice book based on the

Viniyoga method of developing an individual sequence to balance the physical and emotional body, it includes good sequences for both depression and anxiety.

Sparrowe, Linda, with Yoga sequences by Patricia Walden. *The Woman's Book of Yoga and Health*. Boston: Shambhala, 2002. A good resource for women's emotional and physical well-being, it includes an excellent chapter on depression.

Salzberg, Sharon. *Lovingkindness: The Revolutionary Art of Happiness*. Boston: Shambhala, 1995. This book includes essays on what makes for a happy life and many healing meditations.

Favorite Yoga Practice Books

Bennet, Bija. *Emotional Yoga*. Boston: Shambhala, 2002.

Desikachar, T.K.V. *The Heart of Yoga: Developing a Personal Practice*. Rochester, Vermont: Inner Traditions International, 1995.

Devi, Nischala Joy. *The Healing Path of Yoga: Time-Honored Wisdom and Scientifically Proven Methods that Alleviate Stress, Open Your Heart, and Enrich Your Life*. New York: Three Rivers Press, 2000.

Faulds, Richard. *Kripalu Yoga: A Guide to Practice On and Off the Mat*. New York: Bantam Books, 2004.

Gannon, Sharon, and David Life. *Jivamukti Yoga: Practices for Liberating Body and Soul*. New York, Ballantine Books, 2002.

Iyengar, B.K.S. *Yoga: The Path to Holistic Health*. London: Dorling Kindersley, 2001.

Khalsa, Shakta Kaur. *Kundalini Yoga as Taught by Yogi Bhajan*. New York: Dorling Kindersley, 2001.

Kraftsow, Gary. *Yoga for Transformation: Ancient Teachings and Practices for Healing the Body, Mind, and Heart*. New York: Penguin Compass, 2002.

———. *Yoga for Wellness: Healing with the Timeless Teachings of Viniyoga*. New York: Penguin, 1999.

Lasater, Judith. *Living Your Yoga: Finding the Spiritual in Everday Life*. Berkeley, California: Rodmell Press, 2000.

———. *Relax and Renew: Restful Yoga for Stressful Times*. Berkeley, California: Rodmell Press, 1995.

Muktibodhananda, Swami, trans. and commentary. *Hatha Yoga Pradipika: Light on Yoga by Yogi Swatmarama*. Bihar, India: Yoga Publications Trust, 2nd ed., 1993.

Radha, Swami Sivananda. *Hatha Yoga: The Hidden Language*. Boston: Shambhala Publications, 1987.

Satchidananda, Yogiraj Sri Swami, *Integral Yoga Hatha*. New York: Henry Holt and Company, 1970.

The Sivananda Center. *The Sivananda Companion to Yoga*. New York: Fireside, 1983.

Sparrowe, Linda, with Yoga sequences by Patricia Walden. *The Woman's Book of Yoga and Health*. Boston: Shambhala, 2002.

Stiles, Mukunda. *Structural Yoga Therapy*. York Beach, Maine: Samuel Weiser, 2000.

Yee, Rodney, with Nina Zolotow. *Yoga: The Poetry of the Body*. New York: Thomas Dunne Books, 2002.

The Spiritual Journey

Boorstein, Sylvia. *That's Funny You Don't Look Like a Buddhist: On Being a Faithful Jew and a Passionate Buddhist*. New York: HarperSanFrancisco, 1997.

Cooper, David. *Three Gates to Meditation Practice: A Personal Journey into Sufism, Buddhism, and Judaism*. Woodstock, VT: Skylight Paths Pub., 2000.

Cope, Stephen, ed. *Will Yoga and Meditation Really Change My Life?* North Adams, MA: Storey Publishing, 2003.

Cope, Stephen. *Yoga and the Quest for the True Self*. New York: Bantam Books, 1999.

Epstein, Mark. *Going on Being: Buddhism and the Way of Change—A Positive Psychology for the West*. New York: Broadway Books, 2001.

Jeremijenko, Valerie, ed. *How We Live Our Yoga: Teachers and Practitioners on How Yoga Enriches, Surprises and Heals Us*. Boston: Beacon Press, 2001.

Johnson, Linda. *Daughters of the Goddess: The Women Saints of India*. St. Paul, Minnesota: Yes International Publishers, 1994.

Kornfield, Jack. *A Path with Heart*. New York: Bantam Books, 1993.

——. *After the Ecstasy, the Laundry*. New York: Bantam Books, 2000.

Radha, Swami Sivananda. *Radha: Diary of a Woman's Search*. Spokane, Washington: Timeless Books, 1981.

Roberts, Bernadette. *The Experience of No-Self: A Contemplative Journey*. Albany: State University of New York Press, 1993.

Thurman, Robert A. F.; Wilse, Tad. *Circling the Sacred Mountain: A Spiritual Adventure Through the Himalayas*. New York: Bantam Books, 1999.

Yoganand, Paramahansa. *Autobiography of a Yogi*. Los Angeles, California: Self-Realization Fellowship, 13th ed., 1998.

Meditation

Boorstein, Sylvia. *It's Easier than You Think: The Buddhist Way to Happiness*. New York: HarperSanFrancisco, 1995.

Chodron, Pema. *When Things Fall Apart: Heart Advice for Difficult Times*. Boston: Shambhala Classics, 1997.

Epstein, Mark, M.D. *Thoughts Without a Thinker: Psychotherapy from a Buddhist Perspective*. New York: Basic Books, 1995.

Hahn, Thich Nhat. *The Miracle of Mindfulness!: A Manual of Meditation*. New York: HarperCollins, 1995.

Hart, William. *Vipassana Meditation as Taught by S. N. Goenka: The Art of Living*. New York: HarperCollins, 1987.

Kabat-Zinn, Jon. *Wherever You Go There You Are*. New York: Hyperion, 1994.

Khalsa, Dharma Singh; Stauth, Cameron. *Meditation as Medicine*. New York: Fireside, 2000.

Martin, Philip. *The Zen Path Through Depression*. New York: HarperCollins, 1999.

Salzberg, Sharon. *Lovingkindness: The Revolutionary Art of Happiness*. Boston: Shambhala Classics, 1995.

Titmuss, Christopher. *Mindfulness for Everyday Living*. New York: Barron's Educational Publishers, 2003.

Titmuss, Christopher. *Transforming Our Terror*. New York: Barron's Educational Publishers, 2002.

The Breath

Farhi, Donna. *The Breathing Book*. New York: Henry Holt and Company, LCC, 1996.

Lysebeth, Andre van. *Pranayama: The Yoga of Breathing*. London: Unwin Paperbacks, 1979, 1983.

Rama, Swami; Ballentine, Rudoph, M.D.; Hymes, Alan, M.D. *Science of Breath: A Practical Guide*. Honesdale, Pennsylvania: The Himalayan Institute Press, 1979, 1998.

Rosen, Richard. *The Yoga of Breath: A Step by Step Guide to Pranayama*. Boston: Shambhala, 2002.

Yoga Philosophy and Reference

The Bhagavad Gita. There are many fine translations. My new favorite is by the poet Stephen Mitchell. New York: Three Rivers Press, 2000.

Feuerstein, Georg, Ph.D. *The Shambhala Encyclopedia of Yoga*. Boston: Shambhala Publications, 1997.

————. *The Yoga Tradition: Its History, Literature, Philosophy and Practice*. Prescott, Arizona: Hohm Press, 1998.

Govindan, Marshall, trans. and commentary. *Kriya Yoga Sutras of Patanjali and the Siddhas*. St. Etienne de Bolton, Quebec: Kriya Yoga Publications, 2000.

Prabhavananda, Swami; Isherwood, Christopher, trans. *Shankara's Crest-Jewel of Discrimination (Viveka-Chudamani): Timeless Teachings on Nonduality*. Hollywood, California: Vedanta Press, 3rd ed., 1978.

Stiles, Mukunda. *Yoga Sutras of Patanjali*. York Beach, Maine: Samuel Weiser, 2002.

Positive Mental Health

Burns, David, M.D. *The Feeling Good Handbook*, Rev. ed. New York: Plume, 1999.

Caldwell, Christine, Ph.D., ed. *Getting in Touch: The Guide to New Body-Centered Therapies*. Wheaton, Illinois: The Theosophical Publishing House, 1997.

Epstein, Mark, M.D. *Going to Pieces Without Falling Apart: A Buddhist Perspective on Wholeness*. New York: Broadway Books, 1998.

Huber, Cheri. *Being Present in the Darkness: Depression as an Opportunity for Self-Discovery*. New York: Perigee Book, 1996.

Johnson, Don Hanlon; Grand, Ian J., eds. *The Body in Psychotherapy: Inquiries in Somatic Psychotherapy*. Berkeley, California: North Atlantic Books, 1998.

Kabat-Zinn, Jon, Ph.D. *Full Catastrophe Living*. New York: Delta, 1990.

Lewis, Thomas, M.D.; Amini Fari, M.D.; Lannon, Richard, M.D. *A General Theory of Love*. New York: Vintage Books, 2001.

Lowen, Alexander, M.D. *Bioenergetics*. New York: Arkana, 1994, 1975.

———. *Joy: The Surrender of the Body to Life*. New York: Penguin Compass, 1995.

Moore, Thomas. *Care of the Soul*. New York: HarperPerennial, 1992.

Norden, Michael J., M.D. *Beyond Prozac*. New York: ReganBooks, 1995.

Robertson, Joel C., with Tom Monte. *Natural Prozac*. New York: HarperCollins, 1998.

Poetry

You may have books by your favorite poets sitting on your bookshelves. Revisit them after your Yoga practice. In a real poem, there is no separation. There is only the poet's voice speaking from what Jung might call the Collective Unconscious, that wholeness, that union with the divine. Whether the poem rises up from a deep well of sorrow or floats down from the wings of an angel, it can open your heart, connecting you with the universal impulse from which it was written. Consider revisiting Sappho, Dickinson, Whitman, Wordsworth, Baudelaire, Keats, Eliot, Akmatova, Neruda, H.D., e.e. cummings, Thomas, Williams, Moore, Rich, Keats, or any of the poets whose works have touched your heart. Here are a few anthologies and particular favorites I revisit often.

Barks, Coleman, trans. with John Moyne. *The Essential Rumi*. New York: HarperSanFrancisco, 1995.

———. *The Soul of Rumi: A Collection of New Ecstatic Poems*. New York: HarperSanFrancisco, 2001.

Barrows, Anita; Macy, Joanna, trans. *Rilke's Book of Hours: Love Poems to God*. New York: Riverhead Books, 1996.

Faulds, Danna. *Go In and In*. Kearney, Nebraska: Morris Press, 2002.

Fox, Matthew. *Meditations with Meister Eckhart*. Santa Fe, New Mexico: Bear and Company, 1983.

Hirshfield, Jane. *Lives of the Heart*. New York: HarperPerennial, 1997.

Hirshfield, Jane, ed. *Women in Praise of the Sacred*. New York: HarperPerennial, 1994.

Ladinsky, Daniel, trans. *The Gift: Poems by Hafiz, the Great Sufi Master.* New York: Penguin Compass, 1999.

———, trans. *Love Poems from God: Twelve Sacred Voices from the East and West.* New York: Penguin Compass, 2002.

Mitchell, Stephen. *Parables and Portraits*. New York: HarperPerennial, 1990.

Mitchell, Stephen, ed. *The Enlightened Heart: An Anthology of Sacred Poetry*. New York: HarperPerennial, 1993.

Oliver, Mary. *American Primitive*. New York: Atlantic-Little, Brown, 1978.

Ray, David, trans. *Not Far from the River: Poems from the Gatha Saptasati*. Port Townsend, Washington: Copper Canyon Press, 1983.

Videos and DVDs

Ali MacGraw Yoga Mind & Body with Eric Schiffmann. Intermediate practice.

AM and PM Yoga for Beginners with Rodney Yee and Patricia Walden.

Kripalu Partner Yoga with Ann Greene and Todd Norian. All levels.

Kripalu Yoga Dynamic with Stephen Cope. Intermediate practitioners.

Kripalu Yoga Gentle with Sudha Carolyn Lundeen. Good for beginners.

Kundalini Yoga with Gurmukh. Intermediate and advanced practitioners.

Total Yoga with Tracey Rich and Ganga White. Intermediate practice.

Yoga for a Better Back with Christa Rypins. Good for beginners.

Yoga for Emotional Healing with Renee Powers (Ananda). Good for beginners.

Yoga for Meditators with John Friend. All levels.

Yoga for Round Bodies (volumes 1 and 2) with Linda DeMarco and Genia Pauli Haddon. Good for beginners.

Yoga Journal's Yoga Basics with Patricia Walden. DVD. Good for beginners.

Yoga Journal's Yoga for Relaxation and Meditation with Patricia Walden and Rodney Yee. DVD. All levels.

Yoga Journal's Yoga for Strength and Energy with Rodney Yee. DVD. Intermediate and advanced practitioners.

Yoga to Beat the Blues with Amy Weintraub. Yoga and pranayama breathing exercise to help heal depression. All levels. (In production. Please check www.yogafordepression.com for release date and ordering information.)

Yummy Yoga with Christa Rypins. Good for beginners.

Practice CDs and Audiotapes

Breathe to Beat the Blues I, II with Amy Weintraub—Pranayama breathing exercise and guided meditations to help heal depression. All levels. (www.yogafordepression.com)

Breathing: The Master Key to Self-Healing with Andrew Weil, M.D. (Sounds True)

The Gentle Series—Beginner Level Yoga Instruction for Flexibility, Strength and Well-being with Rudy Pierce (4 tapes/CDs). The first three tapes/CDs in the series offer easy beginning Yoga sequences that make good suggestions for modifications and the use of props. The fourth tape/CD is a beginning level II sequence.

Pranayama: The Kripalu Approach to Yogic Breathing (Levels 1 and 2) with Yoganand Michael Carroll.

Sadhana: The Daily Practice of Yoga with Sudhakar Ken McCrae (volumes 1 and 2). Combines the precision of the Iyengar tradition with the heart-centered, meditative aspects of Kripalu Yoga. For the intermediate practitioner.

Soundplay with Bhavani Lorraine Nelson. Not a Hatha Yoga practice, this is a Nada Yoga session that teaches you to use your voice in the practice of the Yoga of sound. (Kripalu)

Yoga Breathing with Richard Freeman.

Yoga Sanctuary: Guided Hatha Yoga Practice for Home and on the Road with Shiva Rea. The Solar Practice on Disc I is ideal for intermediate and advanced practitioners. The Lunar Practice on Disc II is appropriate for fit beginners without injuries. (Sounds True)

Chanting CDs

There are many more wonderful call and response chanting CDs, produced commercially or by individual Yoga lineages. For example, the Siddha Yoga organization produced my favorite calming version of the "Om Namo Shivaya" chant, led by Gurumayi. Try a CD and, if you commute by car, sing along on your way to work and notice how different your workday feels. Here are a few favorites.

Ambha Bhavani by Lorraine Nelson. This is actually a tape, but the CD will soon be available. (Kripalu Center)

Gayatri Mantra by Vyas Houston (tape) A single mantra chant throughout. (American Sanskrit Institute)

Krishna Das Live on Earth by Krishna Das. A collection of live call and response chants. (Karuna)

Magical Healing Mantras A collection of my some of my favorites. (New Earth)

Om Namo Shivaya 10th Anniversary deluxe edition, by Robert Gass with On the Wings of Song. A single mantra chant throughout.

Pilgrim Heart by Krishna Das. (Karuna)

Sacred Chants of Shiva by the Singers of the Art of Living. Six meditative chants, including a long "Om Nama Shivaya." (Art of Living Foundation)

Sweet Devotion by Divya Prabha. Seven traditional call and response chants. (Art of Living Foundation)

Wah! Hidden in the Name by Wah!

Women's Yoga Chants. A collection of chants by various female singers, including Wah! and Suzin Greene. (Gaiam)

Body-Oriented Therapies

Hakomi—(888) 421-6699; www.hakomi.com; www.hakomiinstitute.com.

Body-centered, somatic psychotherapy that combines Eastern philosophical thought with Western methodology.

Phoenix Rising Yoga Therapy—(800) 288-9642; www.pryt.com.

Combines classical Yoga and mind-body psychology, using assisted Yoga poses and nondirective dialogue to facilitate emotional release, personal growth, and healing.

Rosen Method—(800) 893-2622; www.rosenmethod.org.

Hands-on therapeutic bodywork that facilitates the transformation from who we think we are to who we really are.

WaveWork—(877) 928-3967; www.wavework.com.

Psychospiritual process for integration and healing based on the deeper teachings of Yoga.

Yoga and Meditation Retreat Centers

There are many small Yoga retreat centers throughout the world, as well as large holistic retreat centers like Omega Institute in New York State and Esalen in California that offer Yoga programs among a variety of other healing workshops. In the list below are the larger Yoga and/or meditation centers in North America:

Ananda Ashram, Monroe, New York, (845) 782-5575; www.anandaashram.org.

Expanding Light Retreat Center (Ananda World Brotherhood Village), Nevada City, California, (800) 346-5350; www.expandinglight.org.

The Himalayan Institute, Honesdale, Pennsylvania, (800) 822-4547; www.himalayaninstitute.org.

Insight Meditation Society, Barre, Massachusetts, (978) 355-6398; www.dharma.org.

Kripalu Center for Yoga and Health, Lenox, Massachussetts, (800) 741-7353; www.kripalu.org.

Shambhala Mountain Center, Red Feather Lakes, Colorado, (970)-881-2184; www.shambhalamountain.org.

Sivananda Ashram Yoga Farm, Grass Valley, California, (800) 469-9642; www.sivanda.org.

Sivananda Ashram Yoga Ranch, Woodbourne, New York, (800) 783-9642; www.sivananda.org/ranch.

Spirit Rock Meditation Center, Woodacre, California, (415) 488-0164; www.spiritrock.org.

Yogaville (Integral Yoga International), Buckingham, Virginia, (800) 858-9642; www.yogaville.org.

Yoga Web Sites

Art of Living Foundation, *www.artofliving.org.*

A nonprofit educational and humanitarian foundation that teaches a program shown to be highly effective in the treatment of major depression and other medical conditions.

International Association of Yoga Therapists, *www.iayt.org.*

Professional division of Yoga Research and Education Center dedicated to Yoga therapy. IAYT maintains a membership list and publishes a triannual newsletter and an international journal.

Yoga Alliance, *www.yogaalliance.org.*

Maintains a registry of Yoga teachers who have met minimum teaching standards at the 200-hour level and at the professional 500-hour level. It also registers Yoga schools whose teacher-training programs address those standards.

Yoga for Depression, *www.yogafordepression.com.*

Articles and practices that use Yoga to help overcome depression. Also includes Amy Weintraub's teaching schedule of workshops.

Yoga Research and Education Center, *www.yrec.org.*

Serves Yoga researchers, educators, and practitioners, maintaining an excellent online library of research, resources, articles, and books about Yoga and its benefits.

www.holisticonline.com.

Postures and descriptions of pranayama breathing exercises, including the more advanced breathing techniques.

www.yogasite.com.

John Tunney maintains this site, which lists and describes most of the major styles of Hatha Yoga.

Meditation Web Sites

www.artofliving.org.

Sahaj Samadhi meditation as taught by Sri Sri Ravi Shankar.

www.buddhanet.net/insight.htm.
On-line instruction of Insight Meditation.
www.dhamma.org.
Vipassana meditation as taught by S. N. Goenka.
www.dharma.org.
Vipassana meditation as taught by the Insight Meditation Society.
www.shambhala.org.
Buddhist meditation and retreat centers worldwide.
www.tm.org.
Transcendental Meditation as taught by Maharishi Mahesh Yogi.
www.vipassana.com.
Buddhist meditation in the Theravada tradtion. Offers a ninety-day online course.

Highly Recommended Natural Treatments for Depression

Omega-3 Fish Oil
Rosavin (Siberian rhodiola rosea)
Sam-E

ACKNOWLEDGMENTS

My heart is filled with gratitude for the blessings in my life that enabled me to write this book. First, I must acknowledge Stephen Cope for his inspiration and encouragement throughout the writing of this book, and for making it possible for me to live for a time as a visiting scholar-in-residence at Kripalu Center in Lenox, Massachusetts. I would also like to thank everyone who works and serves at Kripalu Center for supporting my stay while I finished this book. I am indebted to my Kripalu teachers who, over the years, showed me that a com-passionate Yoga practice begins with self-acceptance. And I cannot offer enough thanks to my students and colleagues who have shared with me personal stories of depression and recovery. Their stories are included here, though in most cases names and identifying details have been changed.

I owe much to the many fine teachers who read portions of this manuscript as it evolved and offered kind suggestions for its improvement. I am especially grateful to Sylvia Boorstein, Yoganand Michael Carroll, Leslie Kaminoff, Gary Kraftsow, Richard Miller, Rasmani Debbie Orth, Karin Stephan, John Tarrant Roshi, and Patricia Walden. And I appreciate the time that dedicated teachers like Tom Beall, M. J. Bindu Deleckta, Tom Gillette, Kristi Hook, Rami Katz, Jim Larsen, Annina Lavee, Renee Powers, Annelies Richmond, Penny Smith, and Rama Jyothi Vernon spent in conversation with me about their views of the use of pranayama breathing exercises, affirmations, and other aspects of Yoga on and off the mat in the treatment of depression. I would like to thank Yoga teacher and poet Danna Faulds for the light her poetry shines on the present moment. For their loyal friendship and support during the writing of this book, I am ever grateful to Christine Austin, Dena Baumgartner, LuAnn Haley, Rita Rogers, and Cynthia Kemp Scherer.

For assistance with individual chapters, I would like to thank the many mental health experts, medical professionals, and researchers who advised me and answered my questions. I am grateful for the advice and suggestions of Richard Brown, M.D., Ann Brownstone, M.S., O.T.R., Janis Carter, M.D., Deirdre Fay, M.S.W., George Goldman, Ph.D., Dharma Singh Khalsa, M.D., Roy King, M.D., Ph.D., Richard Miller, Ph.D., Mercedes McCormick, Ph.D., Kirsten Trabbic Michels, M.S., Rubin Naiman, Ph.D., Ronnie Newman, M.S., and Anita Stafford, M.D.

For research assistance and her always-prompt response to my queries, I am indebted to Trisha Lamb Feuerstein and the Yoga Research and Education Center (YREC). Trisha manages YREC like an air traffic controller at a major international airline hub—as Yoga teachers and Yoga therapists, we often connect with one another through her. I am indebted to Georg Feuerstein's erudition and commitment to Yogic scholarship. Whenever variant interpretations of the ancient texts stumped me, I often turned to his many books for the most lucid explanation of the point. I would also like to thank Shirley Telles, Ph.D., of the Vivekananda Kendra Yoga Research Foundation in Bangalore, India, for her ongoing support and friendship.

For helping me unpack my guru baggage, I offer my thanks to Ronnie Newman and Janael McQueen of the Art of Living Foundation.

For the wonderful illustrations you don't see, because we decided to use photographs, I am grateful to Julie Wood. For his attunement to detail and his fine photography, not to mention his friendship, I am indebted to Léo Gosselin. Judith Belsham Singer deserves my unwavering gratitude for her excellent photography and her digital production. And I am among the blessed to count Stuart Singer as my friend and computer guru.

I am grateful for the sage advice of my first proposal readers, Germaine Shames and George Goldman. A special thank-you to Yoga teacher, attorney, and dear friend Gita Jill Fendelman, who cross-examined the manuscript with her keen legal mind. I was blessed in the writing of this book by the editorial wisdom of two amazing women. To both my agent, Deirdre Mullane, who believed this book was important and gave the manuscript her close and undivided attention, and to my editor at Broadway Books, Kristine Puopolo, whose fine editing, clarity, and gentle persuasion encouraged me to speak from a place of my own experience and truth, I will always be grateful. I want to offer a special thank-you to editorial assistant Elizabeth Haymaker for her always-available support, handholding, and question answering, as this manuscript became a book.

For their ongoing acceptance and support of my dreams, I'm grateful to my parents, Mickey and Mary Weintraub, and to my daughter, Marlana Ruth Droz.

Finally, for helping me discern the difference between the maya and the pure magic of love, I am eternally grateful to Joseph Alexander.

Page numbers of illustrations appear in italics.

ABOUT THE AUTHOR

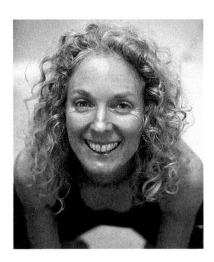

Twenty years ago, Amy Weintraub, M.F.A., R.Y.T., was an award-winning television producer and fiction writer, suffering from depression. Her own recovery began when she started a daily Yoga practice. Within a year, she was no longer taking medication, and in 1992, she became a certified Kripalu teacher. She has studied with master teachers of Hatha Yoga, meditation, and Vedanta philosophy in India and the United States. She leads workshops on Yoga and depression internationally and regularly writes on the subject for national magazines. Weintraub teaches at Kripalu in Lenox, Massachusetts, and at the Tucson Racquet and Fitness Club, and was scholar-in-residence at Kripalu in the fall of 2002. She currently lives in Tucson, Arizona.